A Child
on Her Mind

A CHILD
ON HER MIND

The Experience of Becoming a Mother

Vangie Bergum

Bergin & Garvey
Westport, Connecticut • London

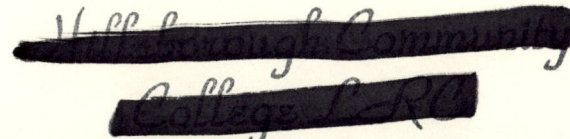

Library of Congress Cataloging-in-Publication Data

Bergum, Vangie.
    A child on her mind : the experience of becoming a mother / Vangie
Bergum.
      p. cm.
    Includes bibliographical references and index.
    ISBN 0–89789–446–4 (alk. paper).—ISBN 0–89789–447–2 (pbk. :
alk. paper)
      1. Motherhood. 2. Pregnancy—Psychological aspects.
3. Childbirth—Psychological aspects. 4. Mother and child.
I. Title.
HQ759.B464 1997
306.874′3—dc20   96–9032

British Library Cataloguing in Publication Data is available.

Library of Congress Catalog Card Number: 96–9032
ISBN: 0–89789–446–4
    0–89789–447–2 (pbk.)

First published in 1997

Bergin & Garvey, 88 Post Road West, Westport, CT 06881
An imprint of Greenwood Publishing Group Inc.

Printed in the United States of America

10 9 8 7 6 5 4 3 2 1

For Sem and Siri
and Brault

Contents

Acknowledgments

This work would never have been accomplished without the willingness of women to talk with me about their experiences of becoming mother. I am grateful to each one of them—for their candid conversation, their time, and their experience. Although they are given pseudonyms in the book, they may be able to see themselves on its pages. I trust that they will recognize their own strengths and capabilities as they continue on their journey of mothering.

The support of colleagues, friends, and family has been vital. I wish to thank the following graduate students from the University of Alberta for giving research assistance: Patricia Marck, Bernadette Pauly, Sandra McKinnon, and Susan James. Special thanks to Jean Ure for her invaluable management of the research process: arranging for the interviews, data transcription, correspondence, and editing. Her generous personal interest in the nature of this work kept the research alive for me. Recognition is given to Susan James for her excellent research assistance, her thoughtful writing, and her depth of midwifery knowledge, which led to frequent conversations about the ideas presented in this book. I wish to thank Wendy Austin, Di Brandt, Marion Briggs, John Dossetor, Wynne Edwards, Patricia Gordon, Sandra Maygard, Marjorie McIntyre, Jeffrey Nisker, Jane Ross, Ottilie Sanderson, Eunice Scarfe, and Marilyn Shinyei for reading drafts of the manuscript and giving thoughtful and critical comments. Sylvia Wheatley has been a spark in getting this work accomplished: I thank her as well.

In my own experience of becoming and being mother I have been wonderfully blessed: I thank my son, Sem, and my daughter, Siri, for being the heart and soul of this work. Brault Kelpin supported me throughout the process of research and writing: I give my thanks to him.

Acknowledgment is given to the Social Science and Humanities Research Council of Canada, Small Faculty Grants, University of Alberta, and the Alberta Foundation for Nursing Research, for the funding support to assist me in conducting this research. I, alone, take responsibility for the ideas and meanings presented here.

The vibrant image of mother and child on the cover of the paperback edition of the book shows a connection in which both are enriched: Neither mother nor child loses color for the sake of the other. It gives me great pleasure to have my daugher Siri Kelpin's painting so clearly capture the nature of mothering. Thank you, Siri.

Introduction

> There was a time on Earth when the cycles of a woman's body, her blood, birthing, and mothering experiences were celebrated and honored. . . . There was a time on Earth when women were considered the sacred daughters of Gaia, the ground of our being. (Mutén 1994: 1)

It is time for the cycles of women to be given renewed attention. It is time. *A Child on Her Mind* explores mothering experiences starting from the words of the women themselves, and as such brings attention to the rhythms of the woman's body, her evolving thoughts and attitudes, and her relationship with her child. The mothering stories testify to what mothering does to the woman—how it changes her. The focus, thus, is on the mother and on what having a child on her mind does to her, rather than on the child she holds in her mind. In a time when mothering issues and concerns are given attention and care, the children will also benefit.

There are women who think the birth of the child should happen at home, while there are others who feel that the hospital is the only safe place for birth. There are women who want minimal use of technological or professional intervention, whereas others accept both without any hesitation. There are women who want a midwife to support, guide, and help with birthing the baby, and others who want a physician to be present at the delivery. Some women feel that they should be in control and take the responsibility to make the decisions that affect themselves and their babies; others feel that professionals have the right and obligation to make such decisions. Some women—as well as professionals—use human satisfaction as a criterion to judge the outcome of childbirth; others cite mortality and morbidity statistics in the evaluation. Some women see mothering as a disruption in their lives, while other women feel that it is a peak experience that profoundly changes the very core of their being. Some women see a need to free themselves from the shackles of childbirth and mothering, and other women believe that childbirth and mothering are important celebrations of their femaleness. Sharing these differing attitudes, beliefs, and experiences about childbirth and mothering is important to assist women who mother to be the mothers they want to be.

Throughout the time of this research (1983–1996) I have spoken with many women about their *experiences* of becoming mothers during the intense periods of pregnancy, birth, and initial care of their babies. This is a time when a woman needs to make decisions about her baby, about abortion perhaps, or about placing her child for adoption. For some women it is a time of applying for adoption, of being chosen by the birth mother, and of accepting and owning the responsibility for their adopted baby. This book is written from the point of view of women's experience: their stories are central. It is a conversation between the women who took part in the research, feminist and other scholars, poets and storytellers, and me. In this conversation I raise questions, make comments and statements, present ideas, and confront my own previously held understandings. I ask you, the reader, to continue the conversation begun here.

In chapter one, Becoming Mother, I describe my research approach. Hermeneutic phenomenology is an interpretive methodology that strives to bring experience to the foreground. By uncovering experience as it is *lived* and by developing a convincing description of that experience, the experience of mothering will be brought to light in an enriched fashion. The central themes of the book focus attention on the meaning of becoming and being a mother: mothering as transformation, mothering as choice, mothering as love and pain, and mothering as responsibility.

Chapter two, Mothers Giving Birth, focuses on the experience of women who give birth to a child. As they give birth to the child, they give birth to themselves as mothers. Giving birth to a child changes a woman, and this chapter explores that change—which I have identified as a transformation, a new form of life. The conversations in this chapter are with women who chose to become pregnant and are pleased that they are going to have a child in their lives. Stories and themes are organized around four major experiences: the experience of deciding to make this momentous change in the women's lives; the experience of having a baby in their bodies during pregnancy; the experience of childbirth pain and how that pain affects them; and the responsibility of having a child in their lives. The women speak about their experiences in great detail and show how they are transformed by becoming a mother.

Chapter three, Adoption's Two Mothers, focuses on the experience of both birth (placing) mothers and adopting mothers in open adoption. At first I wrote about the experiences of the adopting mothers and birth mothers in two different chapters. As I progressed in the writing, however, I found that I could not write about their experiences separately because these mothers are bound together in a concrete way by the child. When a mother gives birth to a baby and then places the baby for adoption she is called the birth mother. Although she may experience many similarities to the women described in chapter two, she has several different characteristics—often young, single, and not able to provide for the ongoing care of her child. In open adoption the birth mothers and the adopting mothers meet and discuss the ongoing contact that the birth mother will have with her child. The experience of adoption, and perhaps open adoption especially, clarifies in many ways the experience of mothering—the fear and experience of losing a child. Birth mothers who place their child do lose that child as a child living with them, but they recognize that they will live with that child for the rest of their lives. In the adoption experience there are always two mothers of the same child, even if that reality is not visible at all times. The experience of adoption vividly reminds us that a child is not owned. This chapter brings out the notion of belonging, for both child and mother.

Teen mothers are the focus of exploration in chapter four, Teen Mothers. What is it like to be a young, single mother in present society? The description of the teen mother clearly turns our attention to the need of all mothers—and especially teen mothers—for community care and support. Mothers need recognition and acknowledgment. Teen mothers, like all new mothers, need their own mothers; if they do not have their own mothers, they need to be mothered by others. Teen mothers grow up with their children and, like other teens, need guidance and support. Teens who become mothers respond to the moral claim of the child, and this claim offers an inner direction that leads teen mothers on a path they could have hardly imagined ahead of time.

In the final chapter I explore the way of the mother, proposing that the response of women to children through mothering is a relation that affects them in complex ways. The experience of mothering, referred to here as *the way of the mother*, can be seen as a foundational grounding of our moral commitment to each other. This is not to say that mothers have a natural moral superiority, rather, mothering is a prime opportunity for moral quickening. Mothering awakens the moral impulse to be *with* and *for* the child. It is one of many life experiences that allow one to accept the moral claim of the Other.

The intent of this book is to encourage reflection on what is learned through mothering—learned both by mothers and by society—so that we can create and sustain a society that is good for children and for the women who mother them. Such a society would celebrate the cycles of a woman's body, her blood, her birthing, and her mothering experience. Such a society would acknowledge, again, that the human mother (like earth and sky) is the ground of our being. It is time to value, again, the human mother, the rootbed of all relationships. It is time to value her strength, her loyalty, and her delight.

1

Becoming Mother

THE RESEARCH

For many years I have been curious about mothering. Perhaps this curiosity comes from my own experience of being a mother and being mothered—or from my fear, as an adolescent, that I would never be a mother. Perhaps it comes from the mixed messages that women get about mothering. There is the yearly celebration of Mother's Day, that honors mothers with cards and gifts. Yet, when a woman stays at home to care for her tiny baby the question "What does she do all day?" is often asked. I remember what Mother's Day was like for me as a child—a day when I would do something, make a card perhaps, for my mother. The tradition in my hometown was that people wore a red carnation if their mother was alive and a white carnation if their mother was dead: I wore red, my mother wore white. It was only later that I wondered, if we loved mothers so much, why did they have to do everything—cook the food and wash the dishes, clean the house and wash the clothes, work at home and outside of the home—seemingly at everyone's, not just their children's, beck and call? I wonder now if being a mother is just a job, a job that one could take on full- or part-time. Is mothering a job like any other job?

Perhaps my interest in mothering comes from two contrasting experiences: one as a student nurse in a hospital delivery room and later, as a labor coach for a friend of mine at her home birth. I recall finding a woman in active labor alone lying on a narrow table in a cold and stark hospital delivery room, frantic with pain and fear. That experience made me want to be sure that no woman is ever left alone at the time of birth. I remember, too, being with my friend as she gave birth to her baby in her own home surrounded by her husband, children, and friends. The birth of Kate was an important event not only for the baby and the mother, but for all of us present: the father, the other children, the grandmother, the midwives, and me, her friend. Just how important, I wonder, is the birth experience in a woman's move to becoming a mother?

Perhaps my curiosity comes from hearing so often of women and children referred to as if in a common breath—"women and children," "mothers and children." There are men; there are women and children. It is women who are linked to children. Where are the "men and children"? What is the special relationship that holds women and children together? We have constructed a public world where men work (at the office) and a private world where women work (in the home). Of course, these traditional roles are changing, but still the image of "women and children" is prominent. Would the world be different, I wonder, if women with children, rather than men, were the major public decision-makers? Would the world be different if men were the primary caregivers of their children?

Perhaps this wondering comes from an experience I had when my second child was born in 1974. I decided that I wanted my new baby to stay with me from the moment of birth. Local hospital practice, at that time, separated mothers and babies for a twelve-hour observation period. During those hours the baby was kept swaddled in a blanket and placed under a warm light in a clear plastic bassinet. Research on maternal-infant bonding was just beginning at that time—suggesting that extended contact during the first hours between the baby and the mother assists in better mothering (Klaus and Kennell 1976). I knew that it would be necessary for me to have scientific research to support my request, so I armed myself with these latest findings to face my obstetrician and the head nurse of the maternity ward. Although both reminded me of how tired I would be and that new babies need constant care—with one person even declaring that babies *like* to be in the nursery—it was agreed that, given a healthy child and an uncomplicated birth, my baby could stay by my side. My daughter was born late one Saturday afternoon into the hands of a doctor who arrived just in time to put on sterile gloves and who left two or three minutes later. The head nurse did not work on weekends, and the agreement posted on the bulletin board in the nursing station was not sufficiently powerful to change the routine. So I was left standing outside the nursery window looking at my tiny new baby. I wonder how many other routines are followed unquestioningly.

Another experience that influenced my interest in this subject was brought to my attention by a woman who had taken a childbirth class that I taught. After a very difficult and painful birth, Paula asked me, "Why did you not tell me about the pain?" I knew that I had discussed childbirth pain at length during the classes—I even searched through my class notes to prove it to myself. How can we teach about childbirth pain in a way that will prepare women? The question lingers. More in general, I wonder how to teach women about the incredible challenge of mothering.

My curiosity has taken me to focus on women's experience of mothering, that is, what they go through as they become mothers. In this first chapter I describe the research process, listing my research questions and laying out the methods I used, and then I explore the central themes of the meaning of mothering that permeate this book. In order to clarify the point of view from which I write, I begin with my research questions.

The Questions

The central question I explore in this book is: *What is the experience of becoming a mother*? Related questions are: What is the experience of birth? Is the experience of becoming a mother different for women who adopt a child? What is the experience of women who place or relinquish their child for adoption? What is the experience of becoming a mother for the teen mother who is alone in caring for her child? Is there something in the experience of becoming a mother that is the same for all women? Or is each woman's experience unique and particular? What does the experience of having a child mean to a woman? What is the nature of mothering?

In exploring the nature of becoming a mother it is not only the outward experiences I am interested in—changes in the body, weight gain, clothes worn during pregnancy, or procedures of adoption—but also, and more significantly, the inner experiences of thoughts, feelings, pains, pleasures, and worries. The only way to uncover these experiences of body and mind is by talking with the women themselves. My personal conversations with other mothers began years ago. Before and since the birth of my children I have spent hours talking with other women about being mothers. It is what mothers do! A mother talks about what it is like being the mother of her awesome newborn baby, her rambunctious and demanding two-year-old, her ten-year-old daughter who is losing a leg from cancer, her seventeen-year-old son who is going blind, or her tall young man heading out the door to high school for the first time. She talks about her twenty-year-old daughter who flies off alone to travel in foreign countries, her son who moves out into an apartment of his own, or her daughter who is having a baby. As mothers talk about the experience of living with their children, they talk about how mothering affects their own sense of self, their own personal goals, career plans, dreams, and commitments. They talk about what mothering does to them.

In my research conversations about becoming and being a mother, I have spoken with many women. With some I have focused on a particular issue—such as "What is it like to have a fetal monitor attached to your body during labor?"—and with others I have explored a broader question—such as "What is it like to experience the baby inside your body during pregnancy?" At all times, I have attempted to get as close to the woman's experience as possible. How does a woman *live* the mothering experience, what is her knowledge, and how is this lived knowledge fostered and respected?

This book is a result of research that I conducted since 1983 and includes the exploration of women's experience (1) of childbirth pain, (2) of the use of fetal monitors during birth, (3) of becoming a mother through pregnancy and birth, (4) of the presence of the fetus in one's body, (5) of placing and adopting babies through open adoption, and (6) of being a single teen mother who decides to raise her baby by herself. These studies are outlined in the Appendix. Many women are cited in this book—all with pseudonyms to protect their privacy. The tradition in research studies of this nature is to identify research participants by first name only. My decision to use both first name and family name was made in recognition of the prominent place given to the women cited in this work. In everyday experience it is easy to see how the least powerful people tend to lose their last name: Honourable Mrs. Jane Doe, Mayor; Dr. Jack Black, Obstetrician; Alice, Head Nurse; and Martha, the cleaning lady. When I make reference to the women who participated in the research, I use their pseudonyms with no further citation. For further reference to the particular research studies see the Appendix.

Most women were involved in the research during the period of "becoming mother," which is often the most intense and dramatic. This period includes such life-changing experiences as: pregnancy, birth, and early childcare for women who birth, and the process of application for adoption, receiving the child, and early childcare for women who adopt. This time is particularly difficult for those women who need to make a decision on whether to raise their child themselves or to place him or her for adoption. There are a few women who spoke to me about experiences of birth and adoption that occurred some years before, yet these women vividly remember their experiences and feelings during that period of their life—some with incredible detail.

The women were located and invited to participate through contact with a number of agencies, as well as by referral from other women. Some heard about the research and asked to be a part of it. The women in this research are ordinary women who live in a mid-size modern city, much like other cities in western Canada, with a big sky, wide streets, a relatively small population including a variety of nationalities, schools, hospitals, and other public services. It is not a homogeneous group: some women are poor and unemployed, others have good jobs and money to live comfortably; some are in their teens, others in their forties; some are highly educated, while a few are still in elementary school; some have chosen to be pregnant and others hope they are not pregnant; some want to adopt and others want to place their child.

To study *lived* experience, that is, exploring experience as it actually happens, I used questions such as, "How did you feel about that?" "Then what happened?" "Tell me more." The study of experience as lived is different than studying experience as observed. The goal of phenomenological research is to understand what a person's experience is from his or her point of view, as opposed to explaining actions, decisions, or patterns from an outside point of view or starting from a theoretical construct. This study is about the variety of mothering experiences and aims at increasing understanding about the broad and complex nature of mothering. Descriptions of experience allow me, as the researcher, to uncover aspects of life that are often taken for granted. For example, when I ask women to describe their experience of childbirth pain, it might be possible to discern when they feel that the pain helps them to learn more about themselves and their capabilities, and when it is debilitating, leaving them bereft and harmed. By asking women to describe the pain in their own words it may be possible to discover more about the meaning of the pain for them and how they can live with it in a positive way.

The intent of most research is to discover a universal or general theory about life. In this field there is often a desire to find a general definition of what mothering or motherhood means, such as "mothering is a historically and culturally variable relationship in which one individual nurtures and cares for another" (Glenn, Chang, and Forcey 1994: 3). The research presented in this book is not aimed at theoretical truth, or at generalities that can be applied to all women in order to evaluate them on the basis of some normative construct; nor does it search for a precise definition of mothering. I have no desire to pin mothering down to a particular definition, because there is no conclusive definition of mothering. There is no effort here to design principles and rules that will tell mothers how they should act and live: there are no such rules. Rather, in this book the focus of attention is on the experience and meaning of mothering in its complexity. It is possible, however, that women who are mothers recognize a common ground in knowing what it means to be a mother—knowledge not always shared through language, but through smiles, nods, and common recognition. Could there be a common human experience of mothering, a soul of mothering that mothers, at least, recognize?

Phenomenology and hermeneutics are rich philosophical traditions that have been retrieved in the past few years as valuable approaches for understanding thoughts, feelings, and behaviors from within rather than observing them from the outside (van Manen 1990; Benner 1994). When we talk about *lived experience* we talk about the experience of being in the world of everyday life, the world as we live it (Merleau-Ponty 1962). Some scholars, such as Max van Manen (1990), have described lived experience as the original way in which we live in the world, the world of a particular culture, history, and family. We *live through* life with an intimate and meaningful sense of its tangible relationships, its language, its patterns, and the expectations that we share with others—that is, we take up the meanings, attitudes, and traditions by which we become who we are. The ways women in this research describe their lives come from the experience of their being in the world as it is now, their Canadian culture, this time in history. In the following section I describe in more detail the research methods I use: conversation, story, themes, and phenomenological writing.

The experiences found on the pages of this book are shown through the women's own words, in their stories. I reflect on their experiences, on my own experience, and on the current research and literature on mothering. I do not look for certain truth, but for insights and meanings that lead to further reflection about the significance of mothering to women who mother—indeed, to us all. You, the reader, may find that these experiences ring true to your experience of becoming and being a mother. Others of you may find that this book triggers new and different reflections. Women who have not become mothers as well as men, who will never have the mothering experience, may find this book useful for learning about the remarkable experience that women go through to become mothers.

Conversations with Women

I use the term *conversation* rather than interview because it better describes what actually happened between the women and me. Conversation is described by Ursula Le Guin (1989a) as the language of the mother tongue, language that connects people together. Le Guin says that conversation is not mere communication; rather, conversation is relationship. She contrasts the dialect of the mother tongue with that of the father tongue. The latter, a dialect we all have learned so well, is the expository dialect suitable for scientific discourse, a privileged language that seeks objectivity. The mother tongue dialect is different: it is used to seek an understanding between people, to share experience, and to make connections. In turning together to the women's experiences of pregnancy, birth, and mothering, I connect their voices in conversation, so that instead of pinning down mothering in a way that is unambiguous, universal, and final, we might open up possibilities of what mothering is and what it could be for women.

These conversations took place primarily in the women's homes or in the schools the women attended. Each conversation lasted for one to two hours. Throughout the conversations, I encouraged the women to describe their experiences with as much detail as possible and to use concrete examples to give an account of particular events. These conversations were audiotaped and transcribed for the purposes of my analysis. The following questions are examples of the ways the conversations were prompted:

When did the possibility of children first come up? Or did it?

What kinds of feelings did you have when you found out for sure that you were pregnant? When did you first think about adoption? Or placing your child?

How did others in your life respond?

What was your experience of body, space, time? Did you find yourself seeing, hearing things, or attending to things you did not before?

What are your days like? At what times or moments are you reminded of your pregnancy? Or lack of pregnancy? Or the child inside you? What is it like?

What happened when you heard that a birth mother had chosen you? How did you feel?

When you think ahead, what do you think about?

Do you think about the birth? In what way? How do you feel about that?

I wanted to keep the conversation open so that the women could speak with as much candor and explicitness as they wished. "Can you give me an example?" was often my only interjection.

In asking women to describe their experience, I realized it is important to listen without critique or censure. There can be no right or wrong in one's experience. The experience is complete in itself with no gaps or deficits. (SmithBattle 1994). Of course, it is possible for a woman to reflect about other choices she might have made in life. She may even discuss those possibilities with me. However, my interest was not in evaluating her experience, but rather in understanding it. To do that, I entered into conversation with the women with interest and respect, committed to hear what they had to say. At times I felt torn by the stories I heard, and at other times I was in awe.

The women participated in the study for their own reasons. Perhaps, for them too, it began with curiosity; perhaps they saw it as an opportunity to talk to an interested person; perhaps they thought they might learn something; or perhaps they wanted to contribute to research in this area. For whatever reasons, the women who participated gave generously of their time and, more importantly, of their experiences, thoughts, and feelings. They allowed me to *touch* their inner experiences of becoming mothers as well as to discuss their outward reactions to and perceptions of what was taking place in their lives. The conversations were intense, sometimes punctuated with laughter, often accompanied by tears.

Each conversation offers a deep wealth of material that demands more extensive analysis than is offered here. This analysis is a contribution to a collective commentary on women's transformative experiences of childbirth, adoption, and becoming mothers. I offer it as one possible interpretation in the effort to gain a deeper understanding of women's lives. I was intensely interested in these women's experiences, but I was not merely an observer—I was involved. We came to the conversations as women immersed in the traditions of our own lives (cultural, political, economic, and historical). This attitude of sharing created a place for conversations to begin, for differences to be appreciated, and for understandings to occur.

With interpretive inquiry it is important to acknowledge the shared understandings that are part of our cultural and communal heritage. As a researcher, I cannot easily set aside these understandings, but I can make them more conscious, so that new understandings can and do occur. My task is to be aware of my assumptions, in order to be sensitive to what is said—to be attuned to what challenges my inherent expectations. How can I challenge my own ideology about mothering and mothers? How can I avoid complicity with my own cultural beliefs that may blind me from seeing another version of what mothering is and could be? Throughout this book it will be clearer to you, the reader, than to me how I am shaped by my own Judeo-Christian upbringing, and how the texts I have chosen (both from the women I interviewed and the authors I cite) support rather than question my own assumptions. The only way I can think of to overcome my blind spots (complicity, ideology, and upbringing) is through continued conversation, which will enhance or even transform what is written here.

Women's Stories

Life knowledge has been lost in the surge toward objective, factual, replicable knowledge as the only form of truth. Stories are one means to recover life knowledge that has been undermined and forgotten. Stories are contextual, personal, and never replicable. With stories, nothing is forced on the reader, for the reader can enter the story in his or her own personal way. Walter Benjamin says that the loss of storytelling as a valued enterprise is related to the changed "face of death" in present society. He contends that people are "dry dwellers in eternity" (1969: 94), who at their end are stowed away in hospitals. While once the death of a person could release a story of personal knowledge and wisdom—the stuff of real life—the hygienic approach to death (in cold sterile rooms filled with more machines than people) has led to a loss of the authority of storytelling. Benjamin's worry holds true for birth as well, as birth knowledge is often limited to Apgar scores, blood factors, and monitor printouts, with the birth itself described as "uneventful" or "routine." Mothering knowledge, too, when scripted into developmental tasks or role attainment (e.g., Mercer 1995), loses the personal and community wisdom that is learned by mothers as they face the everyday challenge of mothering children.

How different is the *story* as birth knowledge! In describing the story of labor and birth a mother (or father) "relates the personality of the child to some piece of the event, makes the story into a frame, an introduction, a prelude to the child's life, molds the labor into the story that is no longer a woman's story or a man's story, but the story of a child" (Erdrich 1995: 45). As the mother frames the story for the child, she has the possibility of knowing more fully her own story, for the story is an enabling narrative. A story offers a personal rendering of the events from a respectful distance and has the potential to lead to an integrated sense of self (Scheper-Hughes 1992; Sandelowski 1994). The story particularizes a universal event. More important that mere entertainment, says the poet Leslie Silko, stories are "all we have to fight off illness and death" (1977: 2). Stories can help us reimagine what kind of world we desire for mothers and children, and can give us clues to create and sustain that reimagined world. Imagination, a powerful prerequisite for action, "can change the life of a people at their very roots" (Moore 1992: 135).

Even more significant than this loss of storytelling ability is the fact that the mothers' stories have been ignored. "Where, in the rich canon of Western literature, were the mother's stories?" asks literary critic Di Brandt (1993: 3), who has noticed through her experience as a mother and student of the novel that stories of mothers are absent or invisible in narrative and social institutions, in spite of the essential nature of mothers' role in society. Is the lack of the mother's story, of the mother as subject, a result of the desire to control the birth-death cycle, that ongoing rhythm of life that the mothering experience so intensely faces? Is the loss of the mother's story a consequence of the effort of modern science to transcend this infiniteness? Is it the longing for technological control over human vulnerability that makes us want to cover up the inevitable experience of birth as well as that of death?

In this book, women's stories are central. Each story introduces a woman in a way that reveals the landscape of her life—her situation and the context from which her words come. With understanding and respect for the complexity of these women's lives, and all human life, the story that characterizes a particular woman's life is, naturally, a simplification of that life. While the writing of the stories comes out of my reflection on our conversations (that is, there is choice in my storytelling), the words belong to the women. Each woman's story has its own unique rhythm. Some of the women read my rendition of their stories and agreed that this is one way their stories could be told. On the one hand, it must be acknowledged that these stories capture only a few aspects of a particular woman's life and may be less truly her personal story than another version of the *woman as mother* story. On the other hand, the retelling, the interpreting, the focusing, and the shaping may make for a different and, in some sense, enriched understanding of those few aspects of each woman's life. The stories stand alone, already an interpretation.

Themes

In my first study with birth mothers (1983–1986) several themes were highlighted—the decision to have a child, the presence of the child in the woman's body, the pain of birth, the responsibility, and living with the child

(Bergum 1989). These themes are explored again in each of the following chapters with birth mothers, adopting and placing mothers, and teen mothers. Other themes are also highlighted, such as the theme of the relationship of a woman with her own mother, a theme that comes out strongly in the exploration of the experiences of teen mothers. The theme of belonging is one that is particularly emphasized in the experiences of adoption. These themes are useful focal points, or commonalities, of experience. I have not fragmented the process of becoming mother into different stages (for example, the three or four stages of birth) or developed categories of similar kinds of experiences (such as nutritional needs, emotional expectations, or drugs used in labor). The themes I have chosen attempt to capture the essence of the whole, to focus attention on what makes mothering what it is.

I think of a small crystal that sits on my desk. As I look through the crystal head-on there are dark spots through which I cannot see. In order to see more clearly from a certain angle, the crystal must be turned a bit. Again, I must turn the crystal to bring to light another point of view. So it is with the themes. While overlapping with others, each theme reveals the experience from a slightly different perspective, bringing aspects into focus that could not be previously seen. Yet, at the same time each theme casts its shadow and its reflection on the other themes. For example, the decision to become a mother could be seen as the beginning point in the experience of becoming mother; however, as the following chapters will show, the decision to be a mother may come before or after pregnancy, or may be renewed many times during the experience of mothering—that is, it is a decision that is made in different ways at different times. I recall saying during the pain at the birth of my first child that I would never do this again, never have another child. Yet two years later, I was deciding to get pregnant again.

Through going back and forth among the various levels—conversations, stories, themes—I strive for thoughtfulness and attention to language, shifting from understanding to questioning (Benner 1994), a reflective activity that penetrates the body and the mind. This type of reflection is "about creating meaning, not simply reporting on it" (Smith 1994: 126). In one sense, it is an exploration toward the individual mother, encouraging a self-reflective attitude, such as found in the question *Who am I?* In another sense, it is an exploration away from the individual mother toward the common human experience of being mother: *Who is mother?* or *What can we learn from women's experience of being mother?*

Phenomenological Writing

Unlike more traditional research, where writing the research report comes after the research (usually described as findings), phenomenological writing is part and parcel of the whole process. The findings are the writing, the writing is the findings. In phenomenological writing, there is a strong desire to provoke new ways of thinking and seeing, to bring about "new forms of engagement and dialogue about the world we face together" (Smith 1994: 127). In one sense the writing is a way to continue the conversation with you, the reader. For all of us, the women in these studies, you and me, there is a certain quality of self-forgetfulness as we give ourselves over to the conversation itself. The truth comes in the sharing together—exploring the shared meanings that the language both reveals and conceals, forcing us to think about what is said and what is not said, to attend to the silences. The intent of the research is to move from life experience toward thoughts about that experience, and forward again toward a deeper understanding of experience, to rediscover it and open it up. Words about mothering are not mothering itself, words can only be signposts pointing the way.

Jürgen Habermas (1987) outlined three types of knowledge arising from particular interests—an interest in understanding, a technical interest, and an emancipatory interest. The interest of this study is in understanding, yet the underlying concern is one of emancipation. The possibility of getting beyond the surface level of the phenomenon to a deeper level than conventional wisdom requires a critical stance. It has action potential, suggested by the questions: How can a world be created to acknowledge the strength of mothers? How can a world be created that supports women with children to live as they desire in their mothering? How does the woman come to know herself as mother in our present healthcare environment? What does it mean to be a professional (a healthcare practitioner, a social worker, or a teacher) who is involved with a woman during these transformative experiences to motherhood? How does the environment influence the mother's self-knowledge or the value of her own knowledge? How are the outcomes and possibilities raised by such research going to make any difference to the women who give birth, place, adopt, and care for their children?

There is no expectation that the results will be applicable to all women who become mothers, that the research will be able to be replicated to yield the same ideas, or that a measurement tool could be designed to compare or evaluate the experiences of mothers. Research into matters profoundly human, as attempted here, is not easily reduced to points on an overhead transparency or measured on a scale. In order to evaluate and extend this work, a study using a similar approach—for example, research built on conversations with women from different cultures (other than primarily white Canadian)—would provide a deeper understanding of women's transformative experience of becoming mothers.

Limitations and Challenges

This book is about the mother's experience. Some of her experiences may strike a chord with the father as well. Grandparents, friends, teachers, and healers share the experience of having a child central to their lives, but I have chosen to focus on the experience of mothers because of my interest in the place of mothering in women's changing lives. I believe that women today are trying to understand the meaning (size, shape, boundaries) of their lives, to delineate the place that motherhood has, should, or could have, in their lives as women and as persons. Sharon Butala expresses this concept:

Women experience the world differently than men do. Experiencing it differently, we know different things about it than they do, we experience *life* differently, and if left alone to try it, we would live it differently. We haven't yet told our stories out of the fullness and uniqueness of our femininity. We haven't yet told the truth about our lives. Until we tell the truth out loud, no matter how humiliating or painful or at variance with society's version, we will not come to know what we are, what is truly our world of experience, and through that, what our roles should be, what can be. (1994: 187)

Perhaps this is what research like this is all about: to discover what women as mothers can be. The truth of women's lives is a story that needs to be told, because women today live in a new world, where their voices are penetrating an historical barrier of silence about women's experience. This is not because women are just now beginning to speak or because they now have something to say; they have always had something to say. It is not because now women's words are clearer; for years women have spoken with depth and rationality about their experiences and the world in which they live. It is not because there is a consensus of all women; women see the world from individual perspectives. There are many reasons—such as increased confidence, support from other women, and opportunity to share—that make women's voices stronger and louder at this time. More women are speaking out to share their experiences. In 1929 Virginia Woolf suggested that a woman needs a room of her own and financial independence in order to give voice to her experience. Along with space, time, and finances, many women now recognize the need to foster inner strength to counter the voicelessness and powerlessness women have experienced throughout their lives (Bolker 1994). Women need to speak their truth from their experience. Ursula Le Guin urges to "offer your experience as your truth. . . . Not claiming something. Offering something" (1989a: 150).

Many women are questioning the relevance of male views of the world for them. Some are questioning the nature of the institution of motherhood. Some are questioning the view of childcare as the primary responsibility of women. Women wonder about their mothering when, for whatever reason, they work outside of the home. Women wonder about their mothering when, for whatever reason, they work primarily inside the home. Even the question of whether to have children at all is now openly being raised. Interests in questions of reproduction are raised by the community— especially noteworthy was the Canadian Royal Commission on

New Reproductive Technologies (1991). It is time to hear from women themselves.

It may be that the limitations of research such as this will only be fully comprehended through continued conversations about mothering, with the courage to rethink, discard, clarify, expand, and deepen the ideas presented here. Such conversations, begun in the company of mothers, need to include partners, friends, healthcare practitioners, researchers, and scholars who strive to understand this important experience in women's lives. The research approach used here is not immune to criticism. It simply is the best way I know at present to construct a narrative that through its mimetic textual quality allows one to relate women's experiences of being mothers in an enriched fashion.

MOTHERING AS MEANING

After Betsy's lunch, we move to the blue wicker chair (Katie, the cat, has gone somewhere else). I pull the chair up and sit with my feet on the railing and watch Betsy practice sitting up. She is three months old.

She smiles at me. She looks me in the eye and smiles to light the world. Supreme harmony reigns as the light dapples through the apple trees.

There must be traffic on 99th Street but I don't notice. Nothing seems to be going past on the avenue. Betsy & I are far away in this warm world. We are alone and connected and in love with each other.

It is perhaps the most perfect time in my life. (Charlotte Elias)

After ten years or more of waiting to become a mother, Charlotte Elias says this poem describes one of the first moments when she feels like Betsy's mother. Charlotte *is* Betsy's mother, her adoptive mother. Some adoptive mothers feel like mothers when they first see the child, for others it happens when they hold the child, when the child is sick, or when they spend a perfect afternoon together. The same is true of birth mothers. Becoming a mother, even feeling like mother, is individual, complex, and original.

In thinking of the meaning of becoming and being a mother, a person with *a child on her mind*, one might wonder just who we are talking about. Sara Ruddick (1989), a philosopher, proposes that mothering is a work out of which a distinct maternal thinking arises. Ruddick defines the mother as "a person who takes on responsibility for children's lives and for whom providing childcare is a significant part of her or his working life" (1989: 40). Yet, in the effort to make mothering—as maternal thinking—gender-less, it becomes disembodied. I argue in this book that mothering is a body/mind experience, which means that while women and men might share in the care and teaching of children, mothering and fathering are distinctive and unique. Instead of suggesting that men and women, mothers and fathers, come to the same experience of being a parent to a child, I propose that there is usefulness in respecting difference and learning from that difference (Kristeva 1991). There is no essential women's experience, no woman *as such* (Schweitzer 1994; Held 1990); nor is there an essential mothering experience: women and mothers are divided by class, race, age, and so on. What is crucial is that there be a benevolent mothering energy (and a benevolent fathering energy) that is directed toward children—a commitment to attend to the child's needs as well as one's own. The need for a morality concerned with creating new social persons, that is, with the flourishing of children, ought to be the center of moral, social, political, economic, and legal thought (Held 1990).

The rapidly changing dynamics of family constellations in today's society makes the recognition of difference and the need to attend to children even more necessary. Adoption (open and closed), step parenting, reproductive technologies, gestational surrogacy, genetic mapping and genetic intervention are changing the fundamental expression of human relationships, particularly motherhood. The questions *who is mother?* and *what does it mean to be mother?* become louder. Of course, questions like these are not just recent ones. There is the Biblical story of Solomon who used his wisdom to decide which of the two mothers claiming the child was the *real* mother. Solomon made a decision. Was it the right one? The question of *who is mother?* has become an issue for today's courts as well: Is the *real* mother the birth mother, the nurturing mother, the genetic mother, or the gestational mother? Where is the child in this diverse mix of mothers? We all need to realize the importance of these questions. What is being a mother all about? Questioning gives time to pause and think again about what it means to be a mother. What does it mean for both mothers and fathers to have a child on their minds? What does it do to them?

It is Katherine Lang, a birth mother, who first attuned me to the notion of a mother being a person *with a child on her mind*. She says, "I've got Brett on my mind all the time, whatever I am planning to do. It's ongoing. It's fragmented my thinking." Sally Corbett, a woman who placed her child for adoption, says, "I know there will always be this little boy in the back of my head and I won't exactly know what he's doing all the time. But I never regret having him. If I could go back in time and change this, I'd never do that. Never." Sally too talks of being enlivened through her experience of having a baby—when friends need her she goes to them, things mean more to her, she can no longer take life for granted. Rachel O'Donnell, a teen mother, comments, "Now, I not only have me, but I have someone else to take care of, too. It has made a difference." Having a child on one's mind is not merely a cerebral, cognitive notion. It is an experience that penetrates the heart, the soul, and the spirit.

The notion of what it means to have a child on one's mind, an overarching theme of the meaning of mothering, includes a number of considerations that will be discussed throughout the book. These considerations, introduced here, are mothering as transformation, mothering as choice, mothering as love and pain, and mothering as responsibility.

Mothering as Transformation

Women expect to be different as mothers. In fact, they are continually reminded by everyone that their lives will never be the same again, that they will "never have a night's sleep," "never be able to go to movies," or "never be free to live their own lives." In choosing to become mothers women worry about this change. They wonder about their changing relationships with the men and women in their lives, their friends, their own mothers. They begin to feel their dependence and vulnerability. They wonder about their ability and their energy. They fear that their bodies will age and sag. They wonder if they will be ready. They even wonder if they will love their child, or if their child will love them. Yet as they express these kinds of fears, they also are assured by the hope that women living before them describe. They hope they will be transformed, so they can be the mothers they want to be.

For Phyllis Chesler the move to being mother is dramatic. For her, the woman dies as the mother is born. She writes, "Last year I died. My life without you ended. Our life together—only nine months!—ended too: abruptly and forever, when you gave birth to me" (1979: 281). An Abyssinian woman, also, reminds us of the impact of childbirth: "The woman conceives. As a mother she is another person than the woman without child. . . . Something grows into her life that never departs from it. She is a mother. She is and remains a mother even though her child dies, though all her children die. For she at one time carried the child under her heart" (Meltzer 1981: 3).

The experience of childbirth and mothering ties women and our communal life to the fundamental cycle of life: birth, death, and rebirth. I remember very poignantly the death of my father at the time when my daughter was three months old. Her presence as a soft, warm, alive baby helped me bear the pain of seeing him move toward death. Being a mother reassured me that life would go on. Nancy Sorel (1984), in her book of personal reflections on childbirth, quotes Jawaharlal Nehru in a letter to his daughter Indira Gandhi after the birth of her son:

Nature goes on repeating itself but there is no end to its infinite variety and every spring is a resurrection, every new birth a new beginning. Especially when that new birth is intimately connected with us, it becomes a revival of ourselves and our old hopes centre around it. (Sorel 1984: 27)

Becoming a mother is more than living on through our children. Becoming a mother shows, perhaps, the route to renewed life through birth, not only in the new life for the child but also in a new life for the woman as mother—for the father and the grandparents as well. Is it possible that as a woman becomes a mother she learns again, and differently, how to be herself? Is it not through relationships with others (in this case, with the child) that people come to know themselves?

Becoming a mother involves a movement from one mode of living to another, from woman without child to woman with child. This seems straightforward. But attention to the movement itself, the movement from one form of life to another, from woman to mother, may reveal an experience that cannot be clearly captured in words. It is an experience that leaves us with wonder at the strength of mothers' relations to children—a tie, a love, a fear that catches them in unexpected and uncharted ways.

In his early study of the mother archetype, Erich Neumann calls the mothering process a transformation: "Woman necessarily experienced herself as subject and object of mysterious processes and as a vessel of transformation. The mysterious occurrence in her body, the instinctual mysteries of her existence, are exclusively the possession of woman" (1955: 291). What is meant by transformation as mystery? There is danger in speaking of the experience of birthing a child as a mystification (shrouded in medical jargon and technological procedures), something women must accept as a requirement—that all women must be mothers to fulfill their destiny. At the same time, there is value in accepting human life as mystery, acknowledging the depth of feeling and understanding that occasionally touches us in ways that cannot be explained. The changes that occur as woman becomes mother, the feeling of a connection to a reality larger than herself, and the notion of having a child on one's mind may seem somewhat obscure. Yet acknowledging and accepting the possibility of mystery and awe can remind women and society of the magnitude and sacredness of what being a mother entails—an originator of life and growth to children, and by extension to all society (Rabuzzi 1994). Jean Shinoda Bolen, who has written about goddess archetypes, says it this way: "A mystical awareness, having to do with being in a woman's body and being part of Gaia as the living Earth, is revealing itself to woman. . . . I am speaking here of women's mysteries, which are *of the body*" (1994: 55). The mothering experience is of the body, and of the mind—a way of being for birth mothers and, I propose, for adopting mothers as well.

Although in this work I explore the experience of becoming a mother during a short period in a woman's life—pregnancy, birth, adoption and the first few months of caring for the baby—the process of change and transformation that mothers experience is not a succinct, once and for all, experience. Rather, the move to becoming a mother, with its relational commitment to the child, is a never ending process. It is a process that is both joyous and painful, one that women accept and reject, wanting to hold the child close and to let the child go many times, at different ages—in the womb, as an infant, a school-age child, an adolescent, or an adult. Women who mother live change in immediate and day-to-day ways, according to psychiatrist Jean Baker Miller (1986). As women nurture and encourage their children to grow, they grow and change themselves. The need for nurturance is not something we grow out of; rather, nurturance, often first learned at the knee of the mother through the experience of being mothered, is something we may grow into, a way to grow wiser and not merely older.

In one sense, women move to motherhood in a linear way. Some women move through the nine-month pregnancy, the twelve-hour labor, the forty-five-second contraction, the slow, painful, passage of the baby through the birth canal, the timeless wait for the first breath, the momentous reaching to take the baby, and the twenty-hour day, seven-day week of life with the child. Others move through months or even years waiting for a pregnancy to take hold or waiting to be chosen by a birth mother, then waiting for the birth of the child, waiting to take that child home as one's own, waiting for the ten-day period to pass (the time when the birth mother may easily change her mind), and finally waiting for the adoption papers to stamp the child legally into one's life. But in another sense such movements are not linear. The linear view does not account for the intertwining of the growing, accommodating, and birthing woman's body and that of the child she carries within. Nor does it account for the struggle between heart and mind for the woman who chooses to give her child to another woman to mother, and lives her life wondering about that child out there that "looks just like her." Nor does it account for the ups and downs of the adopting mother's experience. A linear view does not accommodate the depth of change that such transformative processes entail. So although the move to mother may take linear time, it involves change that is so deep, complex, and dramatic that one cannot entirely fathom its impact. "Having a child drastically changes the lives of most women, opening up previously unimagined new selves, new areas of responsibility, delight, exhaustion, anxiety, ambivalence, and physiological change" says Robin Morgan (1984: 223).

Wherein does this transformation reside? Where does it begin? Is there a beginning? What does transformation mean for women who mother?

Mothering As Choice

Becoming a mother is now becoming a choice for many women—at least in Western societies. Of course, pregnancy is not always a choice, yet the decision to become a mother can be seen as a choice that is both compelled and constrained by cultural expectations, by bodily desire, by pressures of partners, by life desires and career plans, and by availability of knowledge and resources. We know that in some cultures, such as China, the choice of becoming mother is limited to having one child, which limits true choice and raises many other concerns about the treatment of women. Yet in much of the world birth control technology gives women a chance to decide if, when, and with whom they wish to begin the journey into motherhood. Some women decide never to have a child. Some women decide, when they find themselves pregnant, to have an abortion. Some women decide to raise their child on their own, even when very young and alone. Some women decide to adopt a child, and others decide to place their child to live with another woman through adoption.

The choice to become a mother is not easy. We hear about mothers in some situations and cultures who let their children die. Nancy Scheper-Hughes in *Death Without Weeping* describes the situation in Brazil, where mothers participate in what she calls mortal neglect—letting go of the child who does not thrive or who "shows that he wants to die" (1992: 364). It seems that in this particular culture, where resources are limited, mothers have to decide where the resources should go, and choose to use them to support babies with the most vigor and vitality at the time of birth. Mothers come to know "just when it is safe to let oneself go enough to love a child, to trust him or her to be willing to enter the *luta* that is this life on earth" (364). We hear also of situations, such as in India, where mothers may even kill their child, especially if that child is a girl. In a video called *Let Her Die* (Portenier 1994), the CBC program *Witness* shows the extremes (amniocentesis, ultrasound and abortion) that women go through to ensure the birth of sons. It also shows how girl children are killed because parents cannot afford their care, which includes expensive dowries and clothes. The novelist Louise Erdrich describes in poignant prose the intense and seemingly contradictory instincts that surface in guarding a helpless life with the "unflinching eye of the mother" within a social world that seemingly does not value children. She says that at times a mother might, like Toni Morrison's Sethe, kill her daughter rather than submit her to slavery, which is "an act of ruthless mercy. The contradiction, purity, gravity of mother love pulls us to earth" (Erdrich 1995: 147). Throughout time, women have abandoned or given up their babies in situations where they had little choice in how they lived their lives (O'Hara 1989). The woman chooses to act with the knowledge she has.

At some point in her life a woman is faced with the question of whether or not to have a child. A menstrual period is a bodily reminder that puts the idea of children squarely in her thoughts. Sometimes menstruation, or lack of it, makes that question vivid and immediate; this immediacy is experienced should her period come when she does not want it or not come when she does want it. A birthday is another reminder: "Do I still have enough time?" "Is it too soon?" "Am I too young?" or "too old?" Or she may see other women, friends, neighbors, with children, which stirs her heart to think about a child for herself. The choice to mother is not a strictly rational one, where one can just add up all the items on one side of the ledger, compare it to the other side, and get a definitive answer. The choice to become and to be a mother is ongoing, within a particular time and an individual context.

The notion of choice becomes even more complicated when we think of the woman who decides to have a child and is unable to become pregnant, or is unable to adopt. Joan Bell describes how she opened herself to mothering through the decision to become a mother, in a way she would not have if she could have become pregnant when she wanted to. She says, "The desire for the child, such a strong desire for the child, and not just for the child, but for your experience of being a mother, has already opened yourself to the experience of it." But having a child is not like buying a car: even if you have the resources, a baby, unlike a car, cannot be bought. To choose to have a child does not mean a child will come.

For women who place their child for adoption, being pregnant makes the decision about mothering even more difficult. While already with child, the woman who makes a decision to place her child for adoption realizes that this is not just a thoughtful, rational choice, but one that is remarkably influenced by her bodily experience. Lorrie Newton (a placing mother) says it strongly: "I'm really scared that I'm not going to be able to give it up. But I know it's the best thing for the baby right now, so I just keep telling myself, 'Do the right thing. Do the right thing. Don't be selfish,' you know. 'Cause it's my heart that'll be taking over. As soon as I see the baby."

How does a woman make a decision to have a child? What is the nature of choice in mothering? How is the decision to become a mother already a transforming experience? Mothering as choice is not as simple as it seems. Does not making a choice about mothering demonstrate that mind and body are both involved? Does not thinking that a woman can repress one or the other lead to an inaccurate understanding of choice making?

Mothering As Love and Pain

Anna Gurley, a birth mother, told me about one change she noticed in herself. She described how she wept while watching the rescue of a baby from the rubble of an earthquake in Mexico—something she would not have done before Jena's birth. She said that having a baby gave her knowledge she did not have before, knowledge of what babies are like, which in a sense made her experience all children as her child. A journalist, Andrea Schluter (1994), tells how she was caught off guard by her own tears, which fell as she read about a mother thousands of miles away whose sleepy toddler was killed by a shell that blew through the roof of her house. Not only do mothers know what children are like, they know what mothers are like. Anna and Andrea talk of their connection to other mothers and other babies, a connection that mothers experience because they know how much mothers love their children and they know the pain that is experienced in the loss of the child. Women themselves wonder about the love they feel for a child, a love that is so amazing, so searing, so persistent, so fierce, and so unruly that they are often surprised.

It seems that during a war, no matter where it is, many mothers around the world cry with mothers whose sons and daughters die fighting. Many mothers around the world cry with mothers who cannot keep their children warm, fed, or safe. This seems true when mothers see starving and dying children anywhere. What is this pain that mothers experience? What is this love that mothers know? It seems that the experience of the mother is both love and pain, both wonder at birth and fear of death. Are love and pain, birth and death, natality and mortality the mothers' world? The feminist scholar Julia Kristeva states that a mother does not give birth only *in* pain, she gives birth *to* pain: "the child represents it and henceforth it settles in, it is continuous" (1986: 167). Andrea Schluter (1994) tells of the dark fear—an unruly gnawing that awakes her at night—that tragedy will befall her child. It makes her want to swallow up her baby to put her safely back inside. Louise Erdrich (1995) talks about both the relief and the regret that she experiences when her babies gain enough weight that they cannot possibly fit inside again. The mother's ambivalent desires of protection of the child and freedom for the child create a struggle that many mothers face. The mother wants to protect her child from harm and death, but also wants to protect herself from the trauma of her child's harm or death.

The word *mother* means many things. Jung describes mother as the matrix, "the form into which all experience is poured"—the fear, awe and power of ultimate beginnings and endings (in Stolte 1990: 18). Another definition points to mother as a creative or environmental force, like a tree's source of growth (from the Latin *materi es*, tree trunk)—an essential quality of life (Morris 1975: 1527). Mother is life, the source of growth for children. Given such a notion of mother as life, as growth for children, the use of the word *mother* in the description of the Gulf War as the "Mother of All Battles" is misplaced. No, not merely misplaced, it is profane. War is neither a creative force nor a source of growth. War is the opposite of mother. To use the word mother in the context of war is profoundly wrong. War forgets the source of growth, forgets the child. Moreover, war forgets the mother. War forgets the mother who is forced to live without her child. Black Irene, a Brazilian woman, exhorts us not to forget the mothers, following the murder of her husband and the death squad assassination of her eldest and beloved son, Nego De:

My husband could die. My son could die. But I *cannot die*. I am the *matriz*. My children and grandchildren still suck from my roots. Don't pity the young men and the infants who have died here on the Alto do Cruzeiro. Don't waste any tears on them. Pity us, Nancy. Weep for the mothers who are condemned to live (Scheper-Hughes 1992: 408).

One of the ways of obliterating the voice of the mother is through the proliferation of maternal metaphors, such as the goodness metaphor (like "motherhood and apple pie") or the war metaphor (like "the mother of all battles"). Here the mother disappears, is forgotten. But for the mother herself, the child remains on her mind, dead or alive. The mother remains the *matrix* (Latin for womb), the source of life-giving for subsequent generations. Black Irene tells us not to forget her story, the story of the mother.

Some people think the powerful mother love comes with the bodily experience of nurturing a child through pregnancy and birth. Others think that it develops with the everyday experience of nurturing the growing and developing child. The competing claims of bodily versus social nurturing, and the resulting interconnection and love, continue to puzzle scholars. However mother love occurs, it is taken as symbiotic, as in the image of mother and child bound together that many artists capture. Symbiotic it is, for one cannot become a mother without having a child, nor can one become a child without having a mother. It is true, of course, that many women and men speak about giving birth to ideas or projects, which are mothering kinds of actions quite apart from mothering children. In this book, however, mothering actions are focused on mothering children. I explore the experience of becoming a mother through both bodily and social connections.

Birth is the separation of mother and baby—a pain and a love that are deep and difficult. How does the love and pain experience of childbirth and mothering affect women in their move to mother? What is the experience of pain and love in mothering?

Mothering As Responsibility

It is easy to think of mothering as responsibility in the day-to-day, week-to-week, year-to-year care and concern that mothers have for children. Important as this care is, when I talk of mothering responsibility here, I explore a different notion. We sometimes think that babies were created soft, cuddly and beautiful on purpose so that the mother and father would be attracted to them and therefore care for them. But with mothering, especially mothering through pregnancy and birth, a woman becomes aware of the child before it is born and develops a sense of responsibility or commitment to the being she carries in her belly. We shall see in the following chapters that mothers experience the baby as a person at varying times in their pregnancy—and some are not truly aware until after the birth. Mothering responsibility, as discussed here, is a responsibility that develops through reciprocity, through connection with the child as a developing person, and may be seen as a primordial experience of the moral move from self to Other, the natural ground of our ethical commitments. It is only relatively recently that a theory of ethics has taken mothering as experienced by women as a serious source of moral insight (Held 1990; Gilligan

1983; Baier 1987). From the research on mothering presented here, I suggest that indeed mothering does show that the promptings of the heart can be moral rather than merely instinctual (Held 1990). Of course, mothering does not ensure moral superiority. Rather, mothering offers moral opportunity.

Barbara Duden (1993) suggests that the word *quickening*, meaning the movement of the baby felt by the woman, has been eliminated from common usage because medical science places more value on the objective knowledge of an ultrasound examination than on the woman's detailed description of movement of the child within. The knowledge that gives women authority to announce the coming of the baby is easily overshadowed by the authority of the technological vision of the fetus, the printout of the urinalysis, or the composition of the cells of the fetus obtained through amniocentesis. Technological knowledge is capable of giving more and more precise facts about the baby and the woman—especially during labor. Think about how easy it is to pay attention to the information the fetal monitor provides about the nature and frequency of women's contractions, so that the woman does not need to tell what is happening to her. Yet the knowledge learned from the experience of quickening is important in a different sense. Knowledge of quickening is the foundation from which to build a lifelong relationship between mother and child. Through quickening, the mother experiences the child in a way that no one else can, and thus opens herself to her child through her body. She feels in her body the reality of the new life of another being. Through the experience of quickening, she begins to touch her child, to know her child—to be quickened and enlivened by the new life of her child, and the new life for herself. Such knowledge, which can be seen as a moral move toward the Other, is not found in technological measures.

If one considers the responsibility that is found in mothering to be a moral responsibility, an ethics of responsibility, there needs to be a full discussion of what such an ethics would entail. The ethics of responsibility, which I have called "the way of the mother," will be explored more fully in chapter five. The philosopher Hans Jonas (1966) suggests that parental responsibility is the exemplar of such an ethics of responsibility. Jonas, however, describes the parental exemplar as a nonreciprocal relation (Bernstein 1995). I propose that the mothering experience of relational responsibility is reciprocal, that the experience of being *for* the Other—in the mothering situation, the child—comes after the being *with* the Other. Reciprocity means that responsibility is experienced as a developing mutuality of responsibility, where both the child and the mother are considered and valued—moral responsibility is not a one-way affair. This contrasts with Bauman's notion that the being *for* the Other comes before the being *with* (1993: 71). With using the mothering experience as the exemplar for ethical responsibility the body is brought back into ethics. The experience of mothering, of being with child, as found in the notion of quickening, gives the body a central place in the meaning of mothering. It is in the body that women who mother come to have a child on their mind.

What is the nature of taking on the responsibility of mothering? How is responsibility experienced by women as they move to mother? How can mothering be seen as an opportunity for developing and sustaining our moral life?

LEARNING TO MOTHER

Where do mothers learn to be mothers? Women learn to be mothers from their own experience of being mothers. They also learn to be mothers from their own mothers and from their friends, as well as from books, childbirth educators, and physicians. The most significant place where mothers learn to be mothers, however, may be conversations with other mothers. "In talking to other women over the years, I begin to absorb them somehow," says Louise Erdrich. It is "as if we're all permeable. Some days I'm made up of a thousand mothers who have given one ironic look, one laugh at the right moment, one exasperated wave, one acknowledgment. Mothering is a subtle art whose rhythm we collect and learn, as much from one another as by instinct" (1995: 161). A woman (after reading stories from a book by mothers) said, "I've read this book over and over again. It is like I have many mothers with whom I can converse and learn." The stories of mothers can teach.

Mothers learn to be mothers from their own experience. Two women's stirring descriptions of the birth of their first child exemplify how experience may affect how they feel about themselves and their move to motherhood. Gail Lehman and Christine Martin are Canadian women with similar backgrounds and expectations of the childbirth process. The babies were born in large, modern care hospitals. Reflecting on the last moments of labor, Gail says:

Then the team gathered around . . . all women—three midwives, two nurses, and they were incredible! There were no stirrups, right? It was all hands-on! Everyone had some part of me. One was holding one leg, one was holding the other leg. I was held by all these women, and I remember only minutes before the last, all of us just laughing. Them joking about something. It just seemed that there was so much gaiety—that only a whole collection of women together like that could really see the humor of that moment. There was something about the magic of that last bit of time. Then she was born. Who would have thought, who can think that actually delivering a baby—painful, well yes—can actually be kind of fun.

Christine describes her birthing experience differently. She had been in labor for many hours:

Then things got really busy, seems to me there were three nurses, and there was a doctor assisting with the birth. I was in stirrups and they had put the green things on and were very busy, and everyone was draping me with stuff. They gave me a nerve block—that hurt a bit, not really bad, very quick. And then they gave me a local down towards my anus, and that really hurt, hurt more than anything. I know I had my eyes open but I don't remember seeing anyone, and Dr. Henry said, "With the next contraction, I want you to push, I have the forceps on, and I want you to push." I didn't feel him put them on, didn't feel a thing when they were applied. Then Nathan [her husband] and the nurses told me, at the same time, that there was a contraction and I started to push—and that was the worst thing I have ever felt in my entire life. I just felt that everything was being pulled and yanked. The pain was so excruciating, I stopped pushing, and I think everybody. . . . Dr. Henry said, "Christine, push," and I can remember him being louder than I had ever heard him. And Nathan said, "Push now," and then what happened was that everything stopped because I stopped pushing. My legs went straight out of my hip (I think I bonked the resident with my foot), my feet went out, and I yelled and yelled and said, "I can't push, it hurts." I must have pushed a little bit more and then Dr. Henry told me I was to "push the baby out on my own." He had taken the forceps off and the baby was born. They finished with a zillion stitches, I'm sure. And then he [the doctor] came to my side and said, "Boy, I don't ever want you to do that to me again." That is what he said to me.

Of course there are a number of aspects that affected these experiences, such as the position of the baby, the energy of the mother, the length of the labor, the differing hospital and community cultures, and the hospital policy. Yet what must also be recognized is that women learn about themselves from these experiences.

In the first situation one senses the closeness, the touch of women who brought their skill, humor, and knowledge to assist the birthing woman to relax and open herself to the birth of her child. Perhaps these midwives, in their wisdom as carriers of knowledge, intuited the connection between the relaxed, laughing woman and the relaxed and flexible perineal muscles. Their practices show thoughtful belief that Gail could birth her child herself.

In the other situation one senses the effort made to prevent infection (the green drapes) and pain (by inflicting pain), with the doctors, the nurses, and even the husband using their knowledge and understanding to direct the experience, even to the point of telling Christine when her contractions were occurring (information available through the fetal monitor). The doctor's comment to Christine after the birth, even if said in jest, reveals a sense of whose experience was central.

Both experiences resulted in the birth of a healthy, living child. So what is at stake? What is the problem? Is there a problem?

When I was a young girl of perhaps twelve or thirteen, I read Pearl Buck's *The Good Earth*. When O-lan, the wife of Wang Lung, said to her husband, "I am with child," I was intrigued. I was drawn back to those descriptions of birth a number of times. This was O-lan's first child.

She would have no one with her when her hour came. . . . She said no word. . . . The panting of the woman became quick and loud, like whispered screams, but she made no sound aloud. . . . [then] a thin, fierce cry came. . . . She called him in. The red candle was lit and she was lying neatly covered upon the bed. Beside her, wrapped in a pair of his old trousers, as the custom was in this part, lay his son. (Buck 1931: 37–39)

However mythical this description of traditional, non-Western birth may be, it does provide a useful contrast to present Western practice. In our society women do not give birth squatting over an old tub they keep for that purpose; nor do they creep around the room afterwards to remove traces of the birth, like an animal does; nor do they hide the bucket of blood under the bed so no one will see, as they did in O-lan's time. They do not say after the birth of a girl-child, "It is over once more. It is only a slave this time—not worth mentioning" (Buck 1931: 62). O-lan gave birth in the tradition of her time. She gave birth as she understood herself and her life.

I think back about my experience of my daughter's birth, described at the beginning of this chapter. I was excited about the birth of a child, and a girl too. Now we had a boy and a girl. The labor was intense and, at times, overwhelming. I handled it with the support of my husband and nursing staff. I felt good. My immediate separation from my newly born daughter was a disappointment. Yet, I began to think, "Perhaps they are right after all. The routine is there for a purpose. Perhaps I couldn't handle the situation if she choked and turned blue. What if something did happen to her if she were left in my care? Could something happen to her?" The self-doubts that gradually seeped into my thoughts encouraged me to stand back from what I had previously known as right and good—the importance of being with my baby girl—and to let the experts do what in their opinion was right and good—the need to maintain routine and control. This is the ongoing (lifetime) challenge for a mother—questioning whose knowledge counts as what is right and good for her.

As I think more distantly about that woman, me, at the nursery window, and the baby, my baby, in the bassinet, I wonder if there is even more at stake here than originally thought. What makes a woman a mother? Does it have to do with watching, holding, nursing, diapering, and even suctioning? Yes, of course, it is all those things. But is it not more also? But what? How did that mother know that the claim of the child made her arms and her heart ache? How did that mother know something the scientists did not *yet* know? How was her understanding of herself as a mother different from their understanding of mothers? How do approaches to knowledge used in childbirth contribute to the understanding a woman attains as she becomes a mother?

The intent of this book is to keep these and other questions in our mind as we read about women's varying experiences of becoming mother. By listening carefully and attending thoughtfully, it is possible to create a world where women who mother children will be given support and prestige. It is possible to create a world where men who father children and others who have children central to their work and life are given attention and value.

2

Mothers Giving Birth

Through you, Ariel, I'm enlarged, connected to something larger than myself. Like falling in love, like ideological conversion, the connection makes me *feel* my existence. (Chesler 1979: 246)

It is the relationship with the child that changes the woman. Call it a conversion or transformation, something happens when a child, *her* child, comes into a woman's life. Most women who become mothers come to the mothering experience by carrying and birthing the child through their bodies. The focus of this chapter is on women who become mothers through giving birth. Four themes focus our attention: the decision to have a child, the presence of the fetus/baby during pregnancy, the pain of separation of mother and child at birth, and the responsibility that arises with a baby in one's life. It may seem that these themes are arranged in a linear way (the decision comes first and the responsibility later), but in reality the themes become intertwined, with a woman returning again and again to each theme throughout her experience of becoming and being a mother. It may be useful to see each theme as a lens through which we look at the whole, the experience that women live through as they become mothers during pregnancy and the birth of their child.

THE DECISION TO HAVE A CHILD

The quandary of decision-making about motherhood is very real for women in present-day society. In the past, there may not have been any distinct decision; it may have been that one just accepted (or rejected) what nature (or God) brought. Of course, women did make such decisions, as evidenced by the number of back-room abortions and by fluctuations of birth rates under differing economic and social circumstances. Yet modern contraception forces women, as never before, to face the question of whether or not to have children in their lives. Some women try to ignore the question of children; some put it off until it is too late; and others fear that with or without children life may pass them by. Some feel the personal disappointment of being childless, and others feel that being childless is exactly what they want. It is important to think about why some women want children so much and become so focused on having them that other aspects of their lives are overshadowed. One could ask, how can one even know what it means to want a child?

Christine Martin. Will I lose myself?

"We had ten years together without another person with us," Christine points out over a cup of coffee. Her home shows care and effort. The stained glass in the front window catches my attention as I arrive. Christine talks of her life with Nathan. "We always have lots of ideas to come home with, we talk about our various jobs, we know a lot about each other's work, and we can ask each other's opinion about this or that problem, to which we can comment knowledgeably because we are close enough to know what goes on. We have been very equal partners in sharing, both in the household chores and income and in our expectations of working together for certain goals, financial or otherwise." The money they share is *their* money—not his or hers, but from a common pot. What will bringing another being into their life do to this shared adventure? Christine wonders. What would it mean to them?

Christine is thirty-two. Until she was thirty her focus had been on her career. She desired to do her own work, to fulfil ambitions, and yet the possibility of a child in her life kept coming up. She does not want to turn thirty-six or thirty-seven and feel that the decision has been made for her, that she has missed the time for children. In her need to make a decision, she begins to pressure Nathan. He does not like that very much. Could having a baby be the biggest mistake of one's life, as Nathan thinks? The question of whether or not to have a child gives them some "heavy-duty" times for some months, with Christine crying and Nathan uptight. They decide to find a third person, a counselor, to "mediate the decision."

"I've seen women in my work," says Christine, "who look like they have been gobbled up by children and a household and a husband. These women are trying to be very good mothers, and spend a lot of energy doing that. They look after their husband and their children and are responsible for keeping the family together. I've seen women who have lost themselves, in a sense. Everything is for their children, or somebody else, and not them, whether they have a career or not." She talks about the plight of forty-five-to-fifty-year-old women who, after the children have left home, are lost. They do not know how to do simple things that most people cope with easily. Christine gives the example of a bright woman who holds a top role in government. This woman has done amazing things. Christine wonders, "Would she be there if she had children? Is it possible to do both?" Christine puzzles, "Will I lose myself in becoming a mother?"

"I keep thinking," says Christine, "I might be too tired, too bogged down with a zillion diapers and maybe a crying baby, and all the millions and millions of tasks involved with a baby. You see, work is manageable, you know what you can do, you can have it organized, and you know that you have done this for ten years. I wonder about the dependency. It is not something I would want, and I know Nathan would not want it. It is because it is an unknown and you have nothing to compare it to, nothing! I think it will make a difference in my life, but still at the back of my mind I question that change. We know there will be change but we can't anticipate making it. It diverges the course of your life forever, and that is not necessarily bad or good, just that men never have to truly deal with that, ever."

Nathan talks to the counselor first—by himself. "The guy sure didn't work hard for his money," laughs Christine, "as the issue seemed to resolve itself." She remembers walking the dog after being through all that, after the decision was made, "Yes, we will go ahead and have a family." Nathan, on the walk, quietly asks, "Well, how do you feel? Aren't you still afraid?" She is.

Christine is visiting her family in the East when she realizes she is pregnant. She waits to tell Nathan until he arrives. "I'm pregnant," she says, "but don't hold your breath. I'm bleeding." Nathan is very shocked and says, "What shall I do, what shall I do?" Christine says, "Nothing, just let me stay here. You go down to my friends and carry on." She is very upset and thinks, "After finally making the decision, now what if I can't have kids?"

"The deep personal significance of the decision of whether or not to have children *is* the most irrevocable and important one that most of us will make" (Dowrick and Grundberg 1980: 8). Christine and her husband thoughtfully made the decision to have a child but still feel unsure. She says, "You think about it. You *think* you want to be a parent. You *think* that it will be a neat thing. You *think* it will give you the positive feedback that a career can give. But you don't know. You have to find out." The pamphlet *Having a child . . . Is it for us?* available through Planned Parenthood Associations, stresses the seriousness of the decision to have a child. It suggests that women and men consider the following questions: "Does having and raising a child fit in the life I want to live?" "What can I get out of it?" The questions relate to one's job, goals, energy, leisure time, finances, and priorities—"To give someone the opportunities I never had?" "To have a child to be like me?" "To keep me company?" "To pass on beliefs, values, and ideas to?" "To prove my femininity?" How can you find out what having a child will mean?

Brenda Watson always thought of having children sooner or later. She says, "We have been married five years, we have our house, have our dogs, have our vehicles, it is more or less time." For Katherine Lang, it is biological, "a real kind of physical feeling . . . a strong basic urge." There are inner considerations, such as the yearning for a child, the desire to settle, or the nesting syndrome. There are outer considerations, like having a house, finding the right time, and the reality of getting pregnant.

Christine handled her decision-making very deliberately. She wanted a child enough to stop using contraception. She wanted a child enough to hire a mediator to reduce the tension between her husband and herself in making the decision. She became pregnant just as she had planned. It was a rational process. Or was it? She started to bleed. There was a chance she would lose the child. She had experienced, in some way, the presence of the child, so that the thought of not having a child took on a different meaning for her. It almost seemed as if the child was deliberating about her as well. Having experienced the child's presence, Christine can now experience the possibility of absence. She can no longer think of her life without a child. She has chosen. The act of choosing the child changes her life forever. She is captured by the very presence of the child.

Judy Chicago, a woman dedicated to articulating, through her art, the experience of women during childbirth, does not have a child herself. She says, "I have almost never really allowed myself to need another person, to depend upon another person. I've always deprived myself of that so as not to get caught. But I understand how one can be caught by life. It is something most women seem to both crave and fear" (1985: 34). Oriana Fallaci, who became pregnant by mistake, says: "I am locked in fear. I am lost in it. It is not fear of others. I don't care about others. It is not fear of God. I do not believe in God. It is not fear of pain. I have no fear of pain. It is fear of you, of the circumstance that wrenched you out of nothingness to attach yourself to my body" (1976: 9). Chicago and Fallaci, in making a decision against children, do so with a sense of clarity. Yet, something else is hinted at—a circumstance that attaches the baby to one's body, a sense of sacredness, and a craving or fear of being caught by life.

When women speak about motherhood they may sound ambivalent. Perhaps this is due to the paradox that takes decision-making about children beyond the rational. "No wonder women don't hear what mothers say until afterward, when they hear themselves speaking as mothers" (Chesler 1979: 182). Instead of the deliberate, rational making of a decision, which sounds like a technical process, there is a sense that deciding on a child is like a coming to a decision that may not be rational at all. Perhaps it is like Kierkegaard's "leap of faith"—a realization that having a child opens one to life's possibilities—which can only be taken with "fear and trembling" (Olson 1993). Such a decision cannot be fully understood until the child is concretely in one's life.

The Time of the Decision

It seems that Christine and her husband came to the decision when the counselor mediated their tension enough for "the situation to resolve itself." Yet later Christine recognizes that she had, in her heart, already opened herself to the thought of a child in her life, but had decided that if her husband did not agree she would continue to say no to a child. So it may be that the choice to have a child is made before the deliberation, the conscious decision-making, which further increases the complexity of decision-making about children.

It may not be possible to pinpoint the moment of decision, if indeed there is such a moment. The decision may come when a woman is "up against the clock." It may begin in the back of her mind as a girl playing dolls with her friends, as a young woman menstruating for the first time, or as an adult imagining a child at her breast or reaching to take a sweet-smelling baby from a friend. It may not truly come until she takes her own baby into her arms and begins to take care of him or her on a daily basis; or it may not be fully realized until the child is sick and the woman is overwhelmed with a sense of what it would mean to lose this child. Perhaps the decision begins at all these times, experienced through the urge to hold, to stroke, and to nurture the child, with increasing depth and commitment at various times in a woman's life. Of course, there is the possibility that a decision may never be fully accepted at all.

Embodied Decision

Time is running on—relentlessly. Thirty seems to be the magic number these days. "Once I came to thirty, there was a sense of urgency," says Christine. "I am thirty-three and my biological clock is running out. It starts becoming a risky business," feels Katherine. The rhythm of women's bodies may be a trigger to wonder about the right time for having children. Menstrual blood is the sign of hope and the promise of children. It is life blood. Like water, it just flows. It is the only source of blood not traumatically induced (Grahn 1993: xvii). For years menstrual blood was not thought of as life blood but as a curse, something unclean, a taboo that limited women's participation in sacred rituals. Even nowadays information about menstruation is predominantly given in terms of protection, cleanliness, and effort to carry on with normal activities. In fact, the underlying objective is that no one will suspect that a woman is menstruating. Yet menstruation, a blood mystery (Neumann 1955; Bolen 1994), is the outward sign of the potential for children and the continuance of life. Bolen says that if the "fertility of the earth and women were celebrated as expressions of divinity," perhaps then menstrual blood would be held in awe (1994: 67).

The Space of the Decision

Does one want to continue this world? The question of bringing a child into *this* world was a factor to be considered in the decision for both Anna Gurley and Jane Gibson. This world of nuclear shadows, poverty, and sadness causes women to feel fear. Yet it seems that the women and men who decide to become parents see the world, as a space for children, differently than before. "There was a general feeling among people that I grew up with," says Jim, Jane's husband, "that it wasn't a very good world into which to bring a child. But you change, just all of a sudden, and I don't remember it actually happening, the flipping . . . it is more of an understanding of what it is all about." Is this what Jane called the nesting syndrome? What makes people want to "settle"?

This attitudinal flip-flop, this changed attitude toward the world that makes it possible to choose to have a child, makes me think of Bachelard's image of nests. He says:

A nest . . . is a precarious thing, and yet it sets us to *daydreaming of security*. . . . And so when we examine a nest, we place ourselves at the origin of confidence in the world, we receive a beginning confidence, an urge toward cosmic confidence. Would a bird build its nest if it did not have its instinct for confidence in the world? . . . . The nest . . . know[s] confidence in the world. . . . The nest . . . knows nothing of the hostility of the world. (1969: 102–103)

The image of the world as a *nest* calms our fears. In the act of conceiving a child (into the *nest* of the womb) we show confidence in the world as a good place to be, and we are tuned to it in a new way. The changed attitude may, thus, come first: We see the world as a world for children and are prepared to conceive a child. Or it may be the converse: In deciding on children we come to accept the world as a place for children and begin to take responsibility for it in a different way. According to Arendt (1961), this acceptance of responsibility for the world and for ourselves is the essential condition needed for people to become parents. Becoming a mother, indeed becoming parents, may encourage us to take our blinders off, to recognize that this world is full of dangers that harm children. We are responsible for creating a good place for children.

The private space of home seems the best place to talk about mothering. What is so important about the house? Brenda says, "We have our house, our vehicles, our dogs, so it is more or less time." On first thought, this may seem like a materialistic, middle-class consideration in having a child. But what is really being said? What does having a house have to do with having a child? Bachelard, likening the house to a cradle, says, "Life begins well, it begins enclosed, protected, all warm in the bosom of a house" (1969: 7). The house has the power to integrate thoughts, memories, and one's dreams. It is warm and holds childhood maternally "in its arms." Having *our* house gives security, a place of protection and confidence. It may be that the home we want for a child is attitudinal rather than actual—a commitment to be *at home* for a child, to provide shelter and care for a child. When we are ready to be at home we can think of having a child.

Sharing the Decision

A decision without action is not truly a decision. With the decision to have a child, action involves the discontinuance of birth control methods—stopping the pill, removing the IUD, or forgetting to put in the diaphragm. For some, like Christine, it means charting her temperature to identify the day of ovulation as the most promising time of conception. For Katherine, it involves lots of good sex. We know that sexuality encompasses the processes of childbearing, birth, and commitment to the baby, and need not be reduced just to intercourse, but that may be easy to forget. With the pleasures of sex without the fear or possibility of pregnancy (due to the increasing use of birth control methods), the procreative potentiality of good sex may be forgotten. The sexual act can overwhelm us, putting us in touch with a larger nature sensed through the merger and disruption of our discrete existence (Kittay 1983). Childbirth is even more powerful, at least for women who are willing, awake, and not terrorized by fear. "The uterine contractions that are needed to expel the baby are far more intense than orgasmic contractions; and the tiny head emerging from within us remains a magical conjuring act which discloses our continuity amid discreteness as completely as any sexual encounter" (Kittay 1983: 118). Sex, conception, pregnancy, and childbirth are all part of a woman's sexual nature. We begin to see the problem of trying to separate into discrete themes a process that cannot be broken down into fragments. Sex is as much a part of the decision to have a child as of the whole experience of pregnancy and birth itself. Becoming a mother is a sexual experience.

Once the decision is made there may be second thoughts. Christine talks about her fear. Is this the right decision? What about fatigue, the millions and millions of diapers, the losing of herself, the dependency, the vulnerability? How will her relationships with others change? Will the baby be healthy? Work is manageable. How will she manage being a mother? The actual move to becoming a mother is both immediate and gradual. It is immediate in the sense that there is no turning back, and gradual in that the decision is made again and again with each new change. Still, at times one wonders if it could be a mistake. Am I really ready? Do I not have some doubts? Am I not somewhat afraid?

Of course, for a woman who has taken diagnostic tests (such as amniocentesis) to detect fetal abnormality, the decision may become even more difficult. She may have already experienced movement and heard the heartbeat, and now has to choose whether or not to accept this particular child in her life (Rapp 1984). There is a contradiction in the use of diagnostic ultrasound in pregnancy: the procedure makes the baby seem more real and close, and at the same time makes the mother keep the child at a distance in case there are problems (Hubbard 1984: 334). The use of ultrasound disturbs the previously held view of the fetus as a part of the mother's body (with no boundaries); the view of the fetus as separate delineates the boundaries and raises the potential for conflicts (Kaplan 1994).

The opening to the possibility of being a mother—the creation of space in one's life for a child—begins with the decision but is experienced during pregnancy and even further after the arrival of the child.

THE PRESENCE OF THE CHILD

A woman does not make herself into a mother—she becomes one through coexistence with the child. The presence of the child transforms. "Pregnancy is the second blood mystery. . . . The growth of the foetus already brings about a change of the woman's personality" (Neumann 1955: 31). Being *with* child does not mean "as a companion," "next to," or "in charge of." It could have those meanings, too. Being with child, however, is a primordial relationship, peculiar to women who carry within their own bodies the body of another. It is a relationship that develops over time as the child and the mother grow together. It is not simply a biochemical mix, but a commingling, an entangling, an interlacing that goes beyond companionship. It is a mysterious union, unlike any other. Not only is the fetus bound to the woman through the nourishing pathways running through the umbilical cord, but child and woman are truly one body. In spite of the separateness of their blood systems, the fetus cannot live without the oxygen and the other nutrients that are provided through the remarkable capacities of the placenta. What affects the woman affects the child, and as the child evolves so does the mother. They are an indissoluble whole, yet they are two. There is no closer union.

Jane Gibson. Somewhere the focus changes

From our first talk Jane hints at the possibility of some change coming in herself as she moves along in pregnancy. She says, "I never really liked kids. I remember talking to my sister-in-law about whether or not we could be mothers, because we are not all that gung-ho on children, but everyone assures me that you will like your own, that it will be all right." Jane is ambivalent throughout her pregnancy. At six months she says, "There are still times when I am not sure that I want to be a mother. It is a little late now," she goes on with a laugh, "but there are still times when I do not want to give up the freedom. We have had such a good year, such fun. I really don't want our relationship to change." Even on the way to the hospital, in intense labor, Jane expresses doubts about their decision, "I just don't know if we are doing the right thing." But a year later she says she would like to have four children, "with no hesitation at all!"

"We notice pregnant women more, watch them, watch what they do, if they are smoking, or drinking, how big they are. The other day Jim and I were at a restaurant, and Jim was telling me what a great day he had had. I was watching these two kids from two different tables playing shy and watching each other, and was not paying any attention to Jim. He looked around,

'What are you looking at?'
'Those two little kids.'
'You've never paid any attention to kids before.'
And he was right, I hadn't."

But I want to know how parents react to their children and how parenting differs. Jim reminds Jane of the time she came home from work and cried for two hours or more after seeing a baby that she thought was neglected. Jane explains, "This father came in—it must have been one of those really cold days in December—and this baby must have been only weeks old. The father came in with the baby wrapped in a thin blanket. The baby, covered with guck, had crocodile tears running down her face and the father was doing nothing to comfort her. I took the baby, which I would never do in my life, because I don't like kids and I don't like dirty kids. But I held the baby and gave her a soother and she was as good as gold. Later the mother came in and seemed very annoyed that I had her child, and she took it and laid it in her lap and ignored it again. I felt so sorry. I was really moved by that, really upset."

Later, when she is eight months pregnant, Jane says, "I'm not so ambivalent now. The baby kicks and I can see the little appendages sticking out, and that makes a difference. It is alive. It is a real thing. I am still apprehensive but not as ambivalent." After Lisa's birth Jane says, "I do a lot more giving than I did before, which changes my perceptions of myself. It also makes me feel pretty good that I can provide for her. I don't think I have lost anything. I can go back to being the person I was after Lisa's grown up or after she's gone to school. I can go back to working and making money and being a provider when she is older. But I can never go back to the time when she's young, and I really enjoy it. The whole nursing issue really struck me. She started eating solids at six months, so that meant that I was totally supporting her life for fifteen months."

"How do you suppose this change has come about?" I ask. "I suppose part of it is the working towards having the baby—doing all that hard work. Or just the creating and seeing this thing come out of your own body in birth. And also partially because they are so helpless. There is no choice."

Though a woman may have chosen to conceive a child, she may not feel truly ready for the change that she expects is demanded of her. She may say, like Brenda, "It's too soon," "I'm not ready." Or like Jane, "I haven't done enough. I want to establish a career." This occasional (or even persistent) ambivalence and doubt is exemplified by Jane's statement, "I thought maybe I was a little too young to have kids." Jane is thirty-two. Yet it is Jane who puts into words a recognition of her move to mother through her pregnancy: "Somewhere along the line the focus shifts. I can't pinpoint just when. I became less concerned about me and more concerned about the baby."

Being *with child* moves a woman to motherhood in a unique, dramatic, and complex fashion. It is through her pregnant body that a woman comes to know herself as mother. For men it is different. It can be a dramatic and powerful experience for them too, but men who father will not feel the movement of the baby within. They do not feel the hiccups, the flips, the rolls, and the startles of the developing child. They are not aware when the baby is still. It does not matter physically to the fetus how much their fathers drink (after conception). Men do not need to watch what they eat, nor do they experience enlarging and draining breasts. Nobody inquires about their weight or wants to check their urine. They do not have to wear a different set of clothes for several months. They know too that they miss out on something that is distinctive to women. Bill, Anna's husband, says, "There is always going to be something dear and special about a mother and child relationship, such a close-knit thing. It is just something I can't hope to penetrate. A father's love is just going to be different." This close-knit relationship made possible by conception is for most women a lifelong reality precisely because of its intimacy.

The Body *With* Child

"This *participation mystique* between mother and child is the original situation of container and contained," the archetype of the female body as a *real vessel* that holds containment as its elemental character (Neumann 1955: 29, 44). Containment means enclosing: the female body encloses the developing child. The image of the female body *as vessel* need not be a negative one—woman as an empty vessel or as a container for carrying the offspring of the man. The positive image shows the woman as essential participant in the growth and development of the child—the woman's body is the place of first encounter between woman and child. It is a relationship that needs to be clearly remembered and acknowledged. The participation is intensified as a double participation, in the creation of the fetus and the creation of the self (Rabuzzi 1994). The more women are in touch with their own bodies, the more they are aware of the fetal body and its living reality (Levesque-Lopman 1983).

Before conception there is no obvious space in a woman's body for the baby. The uterus is only inches big and, as a hollow, pear-shaped, muscular organ, its ability to house an eight-pound baby is unfathomable. For the first three months, the baby's presence is not obvious to anyone, perhaps not even to the woman herself. She may know the child is there while finding it difficult to actually imagine. She may start to feel different: heavy, tired, sometimes nauseated, with morning sickness, with breasts that tingle and become tender. As the fetus settles and grows, it pushes the uterus out into the larger abdominal cavity and crowds the other organs. As part of the woman's body, the baby begins to show itself to the world. So it is both the expanding body of the woman and the developing fetus, together, that are creating the space for the baby.

Jane remarks about coming to realize her pregnancy: her period is a week overdue, she is taking naps in the afternoon, and her moods are labile. She says, "I was not myself." Women wonder just who they are. This is what Iris Young calls a split subjectivity or a decentered body subjectivity of "myself in the mode of not being myself" (1984: 48). The inner movements seem to belong to "another that is nevertheless my body." The normal bodily boundaries shift—one wonders where one's body begins and ends—and the body's integrity is put into jeopardy. Brenda marvels that her winter coat does not fit, Katherine finds that pulling in her stomach to slide through a narrow passage no longer solves the problem, and Jane cannot imagine where all that skin comes from. When the baby moves, the woman is reminded of her change; when people respond to the baby first (that is, look at her abdomen before looking at her face), she may wonder "Who am I?"

Young (1984) calls this pregnant consciousness a double intentionality. There is a split between the tasks at hand. One task is to have a baby and the other is the awareness of the woman's own daily tasks and projects. "To be sure," Young says, "even in pregnancy there are times when I am so absorbed in my activity that I do not feel myself as body, but when I move or feel the look of another I am likely to be recalled to the thickness of my body" (1984: 51). When women hear the heartbeat, feel the baby moving, or see it through ultrasound examination, the true intention is evident (that is, to have a baby). Yet this intentionality, this felt presence of the baby, sometimes breaks down and a woman may think, "Maybe I am just fat." Anna exclaims, "Intellectually I *knew*, but when I felt a kick that was pretty exciting. And then at twenty weeks I heard the heartbeat. The midwife acknowledged, 'Yes, it is really there,' which answered my question exactly!" Anna knows again of her pregnancy and the purpose of her changed body. A woman's knowledge of pregnancy and her transformation to mother is a process, one that deepens her understanding of what she already knows (Polanyi 1969).

Young points out that women's experience of their bodies in pregnancy is different than when one's body breaks down in illness and fatigue. As women we can "become aware of ourselves as body and take an interest in its sensations and limitations for their own sake experiencing them as a fullness rather than a lack" (1984: 50–51). Thus, the pregnant woman has the unique experience of being aware of her body as being with child while accomplishing her own tasks. This experience of accepting one's enlarged body, or of "thinking twice," may not necessarily be an easy one. The child's presence, through its movement, its reality as a separate person, allows the woman to accept her body with child as her own. Some experience their growing body as ugly, a notion easy to understand in a society that celebrates slimness. Others enjoy watching their tummies grow—feeling the hard roundness, appreciating their enlarged breasts. The body as a vessel, for the containment and the nourishment of an Other, transforms a woman into a mother.

The move into maternity clothes is a public acknowledgment of the presence of the child. Before this outward affirmation, friends and acquaintances may wonder and speculate about the likelihood of pregnancy. But clothes tell the story: "Clothes never shut up. They gabble on endlessly, making their intentional and unintentional points" (Brownmiller 1984: 81). Yet, "clothes have a tendency to deny the whole state of pregnancy because they have ruffles, and bows, and lace and everything else at the neck—to detract from your tummy. It seems they try to make me look like a virgin again," says Anna. Maternity clothes are "just bags and they are baby-fy-ing," suggests Katherine, "I don't want to look like that, or to feel like that." No woman wants to wear clothes that reduce her to a childlike image that could even contain the suggestion of virginity. "Maternity clothes are obscene. They neuter the form and reality of the pregnant women by using inappropriate materials—little flowers, chintz, small plaids and checks, nothing to bring attention to the miracle and power of birth" (Chicago 1985: 123). Do the ruffles, bows, and lace help the pregnant woman feel more feminine, or do they detract from the tummy? Maternity clothes are like a uniform and represent a move toward losing individuality. It is small wonder that women sometimes feel dependent on experts to guide their actions in pregnancy and in birth, since they are encouraged in a "kind of infantilization" (Seiden 1978: 92), to which some maternity clothes contribute. In a "society [that] often devalues and trivializes women, regards women as weak and dainty, the pregnant women can gain a certain sense of self-respect" (Young 1984: 52). Clothes that express a woman's own personality, neither denying her pregnancy nor her sexuality, help her to celebrate the wonderment of the bodily presence of the child, and assist her in the move to becoming a mother.

The Relationships of Pregnant Women

Toward the end of pregnancy women are tired of the big clothes and long to "get back into their jeans." The presence of the child becomes a burden. Anna says, "I'm sick of being this huge. I don't get much sleep. I go to the bathroom every two hours. You've got your right side and your left side, can't sleep on your back. But I'm sure it is nature's way of getting me ready." It almost seems that a woman no longer owns her body. The baby takes over and the woman merely goes along with nature's way. The difficult final period of waiting begins—the waiting for the actual child. "The baby's movements within my body remind me to keep in touch," says Christine. And Jane remarks, "When I feel the active contractions my focus begins to shift to the thought of the actual child."

Women speak of their interaction with the baby they carry—talking to him or her, touching, feeling the movement, noting the movement, sensing the rhythm. It is an intimate relationship that no one else shares. Christine says, "Part of my relationship with the baby inside was the patting of myself, feeling him kick, responding to this kicking, and touching my abdomen." Other people too sometimes want to feel the baby by touching the woman's tummy. At first the woman is confused. "What are you touching me for? How can I tell them I don't like it?" Of course, if it is someone close to you, "it is terrific," according to Anna. "My mother is coming for a visit and says that she wants to come to feel my tummy." Katherine's statement shows the paradox of this experience: "I don't think they were patting my stomach, even though it was my stomach they were patting." The body being touched is one's own, yet it is the baby that is being touched.

Touching of a woman's body, as baby, again shows how remarkable and unique the experience of pregnancy is—being another while being oneself. As the baby grows bigger there is less confusion. It is more obvious both to the woman and to the person who reaches toward the woman/child just who is being touched. Toward the end of pregnancy a woman may love to have people touch her baby, who is now so obviously present. The desire to touch the woman's tummy to feel its firmness, roundness, and the movement of the baby is perhaps a sign of recognition of the mysterious presence of the baby within the woman. "The inside maybe is the baby but the outside is me," says Susan McLaren. This development of boundaries between mother and baby changes as the mother and the child grow and develop into separate beings, autonomous individuals who are always in relationship (Held 1990).

Although the women did not readily speak about their experience of sex during pregnancy, Christine described her changed sexual relationship with her husband. "It is still good." When she asked if it was different for him, he admitted that it was: "I just feel different about what the vagina is for and what the breasts are for." Women's bodies are made to accommodate a child, and the child's presence makes that obvious. A pregnant woman's body has a different kind of richness, perhaps "awe-inspiring," which according to Barber and Skaggs (1975) is a "primitive signal perhaps reaching back to the beginnings of human life." This fascination may be an acknowledgment of something holy—a reverence for life. It may also result from confusion about the whole sexual nature of childbirth for women. Mothers say: "Before you were pregnant nobody talked about sex or anything like that. But once you are pregnant the taboos all go away." Or, "All of a sudden you can't hear this joke. You've regained your chastity or something." Is this confusion an expression of the separation of sexuality and pregnancy? Niles Newton, psychologist and early (1950s) supporter of breastfeeding, notes that in the female reproductive triad of coitus, birth, and lactation, there is a tendency in our society to place special emphasis on the first . . . and ignore the sexual aspects of the latter two" (in Seiden 1978: 91). In the "awe" of the woman with child, there is a danger of ignoring or downplaying the sexual nature of this experience for women. Of course, Demi Moore on the cover of *Vanity Fair* (August 1991) suggests recognition of the sexual side of pregnancy. Will this open up understanding of women's sexual nature in all aspects of the reproductive cycle or deny it even more? After all, the normal delivery room is not a place to share sexual feelings, with its audience of strangers, gowns, drapes, and "no noise" philosophy.

At first it seems strange, but as the pregnancy progresses women experience a changed sense of themselves and their need for others. They begin to feel vulnerable and more willing to accept the attentive support that is offered them through much of their pregnancy. Christine says, "I have felt more dependent than I have ever felt in my life. I feel physically vulnerable, easily thrown off balance." Early in pregnancy a woman often resists or even resents offers of help, while later she tends to be appreciative. It is not just because of a large and awkward body; there is also an attitude change that has to do with the relationship of mother and child. "I'm careful when I cross the road now," says Christine, "I've changed, and Nathan has responded to the change. He is protective of me because of the presence of the baby." But this sense of vulnerability and need for protectiveness is more complicated. Some think the desire to protect may have gone too far. Women are beginning to identify the type of protectiveness that is appropriate. Being supportive of the vulnerability caused by the presence of child, while fostering the woman's sense of self as a capable and responsible person, can help rather than hinder a woman's transformation to mother.

The Due Date

"What is your due date?" is a question repeatedly asked of a pregnant woman. Such questions suggest that the birth process is for the child and that the woman's task is nothing but to watch and wait. In one sense, this is true. Pregnancy ends. The child is born. But in terms of a woman's experience of becoming a mother, the due date is just one moment in a larger endeavor. The move to motherhood cannot be limited to such a linear time frame as *waiting* during pregnancy. The woman is not merely waiting. She is moving, growing, and changing—as source and participant of this creative process (Young 1984). For Anna, "The birth itself is one event on a continuum, not an end in itself. I think it has to be that way. The gestation period is nine months, and I think that with every month and every week you are able to go further and further beyond the birth. I mean, you are focusing on the birth date—the birthday—but for me the further along that I am pregnant, the more I am able to see beyond that." Does the pervasive search for the actual date of the child's birthday make people overlook the growth process that a woman experiences?

The focus of attention on the due date may be a form of waiting that is found in the world of instrument-machinery (Fujita 1985). Such an instrumental type of waiting can be contrasted with waiting "in the natural world," or "in the world of becoming." "In the world of becoming, we can even say that the very way of 'how we wait' enables us to be aware of what has been out of our reach and, thus, enriches and transforms the initial 'what we waited for' " (Fujita 1985: 113). Attention to the experience of the woman herself during pregnancy attunes one to the very real growth and change that occur for women during their experience of waiting for the child.

Space for Pregnant Women

Anna Gurley talks about her changing perspective of the world. "I'm more introspective, have more concern about mankind and justice." The pregnant woman notices that the world is full of pregnant women, mothers, and babies. She wants to know how one lives, as a mother, in the world. And the "world" notices her too. Brenda says, "If you go into a crowded place, a lot of people stop and look at you and smile at you. And if you go into a lounge I find that people really make you feel uneasy, like you are doing something terrible, and you are only drinking orange juice." According to Katherine, "It feels a little odd to be pregnant and sitting in a bar. It really does." With the presence of the child in her body, a woman sees the world as changed and experiences that changed world in various ways. Women begin to question their actions and to learn how to act in the world as mothers.

THE BIRTHING PAIN

Women prepare for the birth experience by attending childbirth classes, by reading the ever-growing supply of childbirth books (many of which are now written by women who have been through the childbirth experience themselves), and by talking to friends, colleagues, midwives, doctors, nurses, and others. In the preparation and anticipation of birth, women are surrounded by thoughts of the pain that they will experience. It is usually the aspect of pain that surfaces in the horror stories; it is the pain that one is said to forget over time. Many women, like Anna, wonder how they will handle the pain, "the whole process without drugs, will I be able to handle it?" Many women, like Jane, take comfort in the fact that thousands of women do it, and get through it. According to Rich, "the pains of labour have a peculiar centrality for women, and women's relationship—both as mothers and simply as female beings—to other kinds of painful experience" (1976: 15). The pain comes from the experience of separation of mother and child. It is physically generated by the tumultuous rhythm of the contractions that open the cervix to allow the passage of the baby down the birth canal and thrust the baby into life as a separate being. But the pain is also the splitting of the unique and particular unity of the mother and child.

Susan McLaren. Worse than a headache

"I must admit that it is worse than a headache." Susan is speaking about the pain. Before the birth she wondered if the pain of childbirth could possibly be worse than the headaches she gets. Her headaches sometimes last for a day and a half and she manages them, so she hoped that labor would not be worse. But it is. "It is just more intense, quite a bit more. When they asked if I wanted something for the pain and Paul wondered if I wanted to wait, I just said, 'No, I don't want to wait.' So they gave me Demerol." Susan experienced the pain as low groin pain that radiated a little bit back into her hips, but not into her back. And she did not want anyone touching her. Although Paul was willing to rub her back or her shoulders, Susan could not stand it. So Paul helped her with her breathing. She says, "I'd look at him and he would help me out and do it, so it was really good—worked really well. And I kept trying to think about the baby coming out, that it (the cervix) is just opening up, that the pain is good. I kept trying to think it was positive."

Susan and Paul waited so long for this baby. Although only married for three years, it seemed to Susan that having a child would just never happen. In fact, it was through having a uterine lining biopsy that Susan found out she was pregnant. She could not believe it! "The only thing I had noticed, and this had happened to me one other time, was that my breasts were really very, terribly sore—like I couldn't run around, you know, couldn't go up and down the stairs. But this had happened once before and, oh no, I wasn't pregnant. So when it happened this time, I was so fed up with my body not doing things right, that I thought, well, I'm not pregnant. I have a feeling, now, that I might have been pregnant before—but I don't know.

"It is really funny, I have always thought that pregnant ladies looked really great. It is not that I don't like how I look, but I am somewhat self-conscious at times. I want people to know that I am pregnant and not fat. And we went to a dance and I was wearing a sort of loose dress, and I felt funny dancing. I don't know why. It is not like I am humongous, you know, it was just sort of . . . I guess I felt a little self-conscious dancing."

The children in her grade one class are interested in her changing shape. Susan heard two little boys at the back of the room,

"I think she is having a baby."

"No, she is not. She is getting fatter."

"She isn't. She is not getting fat because getting fat is not a nice thing to say about ladies."

"I really watch it," says Susan, "I feel guilty when I don't have my veggies for the day. But I also feel a little rebellious. There seems to be so much pressure from people that you have to do this, you have to do this, you have to do that—'How can you deprive your child?' I have quit drinking, and no coffee. I had a can of Pepsi, and someone reminded me of the amount of caffeine in that, or I accidentally stood in front of the microwave, and it was 'Oh my god, what are you doing standing in front of the microwave?' It is almost to the point where, 'for goodness sake, guys, you know, one cup of coffee is not going to deform my child, or a half a beer.' It has gone to the extreme."

Early in her pregnancy Susan was concerned that she would not be able to stand up to her doctor, or that she would get worried if things were not happening when everyone says they should. She seemed to be more vulnerable than usual. For example, she wanted to change her doctor because she had heard that some of the doctors he worked with were "butcher types," who did episiotomies ending up "at your knee-caps!" "Butcher types is how they were described," says Susan. "Well, I literally went into a panic. So I brought up my concern about who I would have if he wasn't there and he sort of gave me the go ahead, so I changed. I panic a lot, I'm scared of walking, slipping on the ice, and driving when it is really snowy. I've always been gutsy, it never bothered me."

When Susan talks about the pain, she really is concerned that she has not been too noisy and that she has been good, that is, not "out of control." "I just didn't want to be yelling, and it was hard to judge how loud you are. It was such a relief at that point to finally start pushing," Susan admits. "They thought he'd be out a lot faster but the cervix was not retracting, so eventually the doctor decided to use forceps. So he gave me the needles, we got pushing again, and I could feel where he was pulling—and there was suddenly a click, and he says, 'Well, you're doing it yourself now.' The baby was born at a quarter after eleven and then I couldn't believe the sensation because it was . . . as soon as I saw him, it was as if everything was gone. It gets very blurry. I guess it was unpleasant for a while. But it was a nice feeling that it was over. It was just mostly feeling him and seeing him.

"I think it was a useful experience," says Susan. "I would go through it again. I have no hesitation about that. And at the time I kept thinking that this is for the baby. I learned a lot more about Paul. We both said afterward that it was a love-deepening thing. I think that is one of the best things of the whole labor. And I learned about myself. I've gone through other painful situations. I was married before and for a time I thought this was it, that I couldn't survive anymore. And now I look back at it and realize it was a positive growth situation for me. I look back on myself and can't believe how I used to be."

One wonders if there is something important in the pangs of childbirth that is true for all women—those who pleasure in its labor, those who endure, and those who suffer. Some births are short and intense, some long and exhausting, and some need medical intervention and treatment with forceps, medication, and cesarean delivery. Christine experienced intense, excruciating pain (partly due to the use of forceps) and yet two months later says, "I'm glad I didn't miss it and I would wish other women could experience it." Then she pauses and wonders, "Why did I say that?" She goes on:

I don't think one should focus on the pain, that women should have to experience pain. But in the pain there is an experience of being inward and involved in feeling the pain—not enjoying it but taking hold, enduring, or whatever you do to handle it—and knowing that it is going to produce a child. That is what it is, not to focus on the pain, but to see what the pain does to you, how it changes you.

Is it possible that the separation from the child inside one's body, with its accompanying pain, is a penetrating aspect of a woman's transformation to mother? Is it possible that the pain helps one recognize the profoundness of the mother-child connection?

Can Birthing Pain Be Described?

In order to explore the nature of birthing pain, it is important to let go, for a moment at least, of some of our current assumptions and beliefs:

Pain Should Be Denied. Some childbirth educators think that by removing the word "pain" from the language of birthing, they will prepare women to take a more positive posture and to accept more readily the challenge and joy of the birth. Some talk of contractions, others refer to rushes or discomfort when they actually mean *pain*. Anna talks about her expectation: "Early in pregnancy I had felt that I was not going to see this as a painful experience, I was going to relax, and go with the flow, but after having listened to a tape of a woman in labor, and hearing about transition, and how disoriented you become—a very tough time—really dispelled any notions that there would be no pain. Pain really does exist." While a woman's positive attitude is important, denial of pain may create expectations not borne out in reality. What is being denied in the denial of birthing pain?

Pain Must Be Relieved. The belief that pain must be relieved pervades our society, from the advertisement of over-the-counter drugs to the medical need to "give something for the pain." Rich (1976: 152) suggests that this notion "is a dangerous mechanism, which can cause us to lose touch not just with our painful sensations but with ourselves." Could it be that the fear and anxiety of pain stands in the way of drawing on the fundamental source of life and spirit women have? What is taken away in attempting to take away the pain of giving birth?

Pain Is Only Negative. Childbirth pain is a normal accompaniment of birthing and may arise from dilation of the cervix, the contraction and distension of the uterus, distension of the outlet, vulva, and perineum, and from factors such as pain-sensitive structures in the pelvis (Bonica 1975). Birthing pain brings life. The fact that childbirth is now primarily a medical event, occurring in an atmosphere associated with sickness and death, supports the underlying notion that the pregnancy-birth event is a disease condition. In a nursing text on pain (Meinhart and McCaffery 1983), labor pain is included in the chapter on pain syndromes along with phantom limb pain, arthritis, headache, and pain syndromes associated with cancer. The term *syndrome* is defined as "a group of signs and symptoms that collectively indicate or characterize disease, psychological disorder, or other abnormal conditions" (Morris 1975: 1305).

There is a danger in romanticizing pain. We know childbirth and its pain has taken its toll, with death and horror so vividly described in medical case histories as well as biographies and novels. It is small wonder that women welcome prescribed anesthesia, believing it will mean less pain and danger at birth (Hubbard 1984: 338). At one level pain is a sign of distress and possible danger; yet birthing pain can be normal, and with the pain comes life. Can birthing pain be shown to be a positive, normal experience?

Pain Is Punishment. The word *pain* derives from the Greek *poinē,* meaning penalty. This origin is suggestive of the notion that women are being punished for the "crime" of pregnancy or, symbolically, for tasting of the tree of knowledge, that is, "knowing too much" (Seiden 1978: 95). Is it possible that the nonacceptance or fear of pain comes from women's nonacceptance of, or alienation from their bodies, leading to fear of helplessness, of dependence, and of inappropriate behavior? Rather than accepting the notion that childbirth pain is a punishment to be mutely endured, one wonders if women could be seen to acknowledge their physicality, their passion, their sexuality, their whole female existence. Yet even here there are limits between ennobling pain and self-destructive hurtful pain. But can giving birth be an event of proud endurance of pain in the service of a desired goal, not unlike contact and endurance sports (Seiden 1978: 101)? Can birthing pain be seen as an opportunity and a challenge?

Pain Can Be Explained. There are theories that explain childbirth pain physically, psychologically, sociologically, and culturally. These theories and explanations contribute to our understanding of pain, but they also fragment the sense of wholeness of the pain experience. When we explain, we stand apart from the phenomenon and observe, trying to fit everything into systematic order. Exploring the phenomenon of birthing pain is an attempt to grasp that primordial wholeness of the experienced pain—the participation of women in their pain. Is there experiential wholeness within the nature of women's birthing pain?

Birthing pain, like other pain, is difficult to describe. "Its resistance to language is not simply one of its incidental or accidental attributes but is essential to what it is," says Elaine Scarry. "This resistance to language is because physical pain, unlike any other state of consciousness—has no referential content. It is not of or for anything" (1985: 5). But here we need to look again. The pain of childbirth is different from the enveloping effects of other pain: "these pains one could follow with one's mind" (Margaret Mead, in Sorel 1984: 339). And birthing pain produces a child. However violent and terrible the pains are, this connection needs to be remembered: "You get a prize in the end. You've accomplished something that you can look back and say, 'Gee, I did that,' " says Susan. If birthing pain is likened to the pain of mountain climbing, the pain of running the last few yards of an Olympic race, the pain of the downhill skier in search of the gold medal, rather than the pain of arthritis, cancer, or other illness (Melzack, Taenzer, Feldman, & Kinch 1980), will that change women's preparation for and attitude about the pain? Childbirth pain is of and for the child, and in this fact is contained the possibility of personal good. "I did that," or as Paula Peters says, "I can do anything now."

But still it is hard to find the right words. Women say the pain is powerful, intense, overwhelming, cramp-like, stretching, burning, pressuring, tiring, and exhausting. They say:

I withdrew into myself, had few thoughts. (Helen Crozier)

I was immersed in a physical sensation; lost awareness of time and what was going on around me. (Victoria LeClair)

I feared that I wouldn't be able to stand the pain—would lose control of myself—maybe even die. (Paula Peters)

I was brought to the core of myself. I was pitted against myself. (Iris Cummings)

It was definitely, definitely painful. When she crowned, it hurt a lot. I can't deny that. But as each hour passes the memory gets less pronounced. And look what I have to show for it. . . . [Seven months later] I've almost forgotten, am surprised how easy it was. (Anna Gurley)

I have a picture in my mind's eye of being in pain, but I can't remember the pain. (Laura Brown)

After the birth I almost had a feeling that perhaps I imagined the pain. Was it really as hard as I thought it was? (Paula Peters)

"Who can remember pain once it is over?" writes Atwood. "All that remains of it is a shadow, not in the mind even, in the flesh. Pain marks you, but too deep to see" (1985: 135).

I Am My Painful Body

"I had my first contraction in the bathroom. It came from nowhere—an internal tornado picked up and hurled every organ toward my skin but nothing showed outwardly; the force was wholly absorbed. I couldn't recognize my own body in pain" (Israeloff 1982: 86–87). Childbirth pain is something deep and powerful. There is the localized, surface pain, such as the burning and stinging as the tissue stretches to release the baby's head, yet at the same time there is that deep inner pain that expresses itself as "being in pain." The inwardness of childbirth pain is experienced through a feeling of unreality, of being in a fog; or a sense that time has stopped, is going on forever, is irrelevant. There is little awareness of the people around. "I don't remember what was talked about. I was totally inward" (Iris Cummings). The origin of the word "birth," from the Old Norse *burdhr*, means "to carry," "to bear children." As a woman, I am this body, I am this pain. The Old English word for birth, *forberan* means "enduring." To bear, to carry on, to endure the pain is a part of the birth experience. Pain is experienced by one's stance in relation to it—as a woman of autonomy and personal power or as a woman at the mercy of the environment or the doctor, alienated from her body and subject to fearful thoughts and imaginings. As women accept and take hold of their power to—both figuratively and literally—"stand up" and actively birth their own children rather than be delivered, as in the vulnerable "lying on one's back" position, they do not deny the pain but carry it.

Women are empowered by their way of standing in relationship to pain-as-experienced: their riding with it and enduring it, or their being overwhelmed by it. Both enduring and suffering are experienced by women. In the attention given to the pain there is a realization that the pain is not static and unchanging but dynamic and moving, and that the power of attention can become a key factor in working with and lessening the pain. By focusing attention inwardly, we can gain a better understanding of the numerous signals our bodies transmit regarding what to do to help ourselves through the pain (Heckler 1984: 61). The universal acceptance of Cartesian philosophy, which separates the mind and locates selfhood with the "thinking thing," *res cogitans*, has invaded our thought to such an extent that we risk losing touch with our body wisdom, the "material being," *res extensa*. In childbirth, pain embodiment—understood in the notion "I am my body"—becomes a concrete reality not to be ignored. Yet the regular, intense, continuous contractions take their toll of energy and resources. Exhausted with the pain of fatigue, the feeling is one of "I just cannot go on." The exertion does not involve just the physical power of the uterus or the intellectual power of the mind, but the unity of self that calls women to use all their resources. Women carry on. Of course, there is no other option. There is no turning back.

The pain of labor demands action: grunting, screaming, walking, finding a comfortable position, active relaxation, breathing patterns, focusing attention, or having a bath. Women say things like: "I didn't know what to do and needed someone to help me" (Xavier Marshall); "I tried to find a comfortable position, was impatient, angry, and shaking" (Flo Hammer); or "I screamed, or wanted to scream, to bite on something. I cried because it hurt so much" (Ellie Robertson). We need to ask, "What can be done to assist?"

The Australian myth of Eingana (the Great Earth Mother, fertility herself, the source of all life) gives a clue to the birth cry: "Eingana's travail to give birth is also the explanation of the sound made by the bull-roarer in the Kunapappi ritual. . . . Eingana was rolling about, every way, on the ground. She was groaning and calling out . . . making a big noise" (Meltzer 1981: 11). Anna talks about the "primal, guttural kind of noise that came when pushing, and the whinnying noise while crowning. Making the noise helped the effort, it seemed." Earlier in labor there may be moments of laughing. Crying, laughing, the bull's roar, the screams, the whinnying, all express the woman's experience of the pain and the intensity of labor. She may not even be entirely conscious that the sound is coming from herself (Barber and Skaggs 1975). Giving voice to women's pain in childbirth assists their use of the pain experience to express themselves and the reality of their world. It transforms women's experience of pain into something useful to them. Nonetheless, pain should not be stoically endured by women for some psychological or physiological value (Meinhardt and McCaffery 1983). By giving voice to pain, women help themselves through it. They can use the pain to express themselves rather than let the pain defeat them, belittle them, or leave them feeling helpless and angry.

In 1884 Doctor Engelmann, in an ethnographic account of laboring women from various cultures, wrote, "The parturient must be guided by her own actions, and in a position assumed by her own comfort and by the dictates of her instinct. . . . The recumbent position retards labour and is inimical to easy, safe, and rapid delivery" (1884: 149). Nearly a hundred years later, after the recumbent position had been used almost routinely by obstetricians, another doctor, Odent, harkens back to the instinctual knowledge of the body. "These last years, we understand better and better what to do to help the mother become more instinctive, to forget what is cultural, to reduce the control of the neocortex, to change her level of consciousness so that the labour seems to be easier" (Odent 1981: 9). If women obey their own impulses and become more instinctual, they may assume a squatting, kneeling, or sitting posture. "This would . . . often do away with the necessity of resorting to the forceps, which, though a great blessing, too often become the reverse in the hands of eager obstetricians, who are inclined to use them on the least occasion, or without any real occasion at all" (Engelmann 1884: 149).

Christine, in discussing the best position for labor with her doctor, found that he agreed that squatting is the best one, because the birth canal is not straight down but curved. So "you need to squat." But in her labor Christine had only two choices, the delivery table or the birthing chair, as the hospital is not set up to handle the squatting position, which requires someone to assist. At home it was different, as Anna describes, "When I wanted to push Bill helped me get into a squatting position. I found that really good, and I had no trouble pushing—a very primal feeling. Betty [a friend] and Mary [her mother-in-law] came and got on either side of me and I could just kind of lean on them." Finding a good position helps the woman to deal with the pain.

Space for Pain

There is not much tolerance for pain in everyday life. We try to remove pain as quickly as we can with drugs, with entertainment, with sex, with divorce, or with technology. Anna says, "I don't think society allows us to deal with the harsher realities of life, and I don't think we are better off for it. . . . What we lose is the intensity of living—a vitality, the risk of being hurt or the risk of the responsibility of friendship and all that is involved in that." But surely life should not be harsher. Surely, we have enough pain.

How can women experience the pain of birthing in a way that fosters personal growth without suffering unnecessarily? How can pain serve the process of becoming a mother rather than debilitate or cause "residual maternal and psychological problems," which, according to Meinhardt and McCaffery (1983: 37), result from severe pain? How can the space in which women give birth aid them to transform their experience of pain into something useful for their lives?

Women want to be good during labor. "I was really worried that I was being really noisy. I didn't want to be yelling, and then it's hard to judge how loud you are," says Susan. To be good often means not to make too much noise, to be cooperative, and not to make a scene. In their effort to be good, to please hospital staff, are women required to fit some predesigned criteria of what is appropriate behavior? In their effort to be good, do women deny the potential they have to help themselves through the pain?

Susan and Jane gave birth in the birthing room, the hospital space that has been designed to humanize obstetrical care by providing a more comfortable, restful, private environment—generally furnished with curtains, carpets, an easy chair, a coffee table, a telephone, a television, and a bed. The birthing room concept allows for the woman to labor and deliver in the same room, as opposed to moving from one room to another at the beginning of the birth itself. One often hears the term *homelike* in reference to the birthing room. Do not the carpeted floor, the piped-in music, the bedside television, and the handy telephone sound more like a motel than a home? One then wonders whose home the birthing room is like—the doctor's, the nurse's, the birthing woman's, or the traveler's? What does it mean to be at home? To be at home is to be at ease, unconstrained and unembarrassed, familiar, and so on. To be at home is to be ourselves with no need to explain or play games, no guard against the misconceptions of others, and no fear of abandonment. In such an environment, one does not worry about being good—in fact, one does not even think about the need to be good or to be cooperative. Christine says, "I can remember complaining that I didn't want to cooperate." Perhaps the question needs to be asked, what did it mean for Christine to feel that she needed to cooperate? If the woman is at home, where she is the center of the action, the central figure in the act of birthing her child, then it is the people surrounding her who need to cooperate with her. "Unless the woman has some psychiatric disorder impairing her competence for decision making . . . she should have, as nearly as possible, the same degree of control over her activities and companions as she has in her own home" (Seiden 1978: 101). Being in her own home, Paula says, "I feel I rode the contractions in the sense of expressing what they felt like to me at the time—felt comfortable about being spontaneous in both vocal and physical reactions. Being home felt right." She did what was right for her and her companions cooperated with her. What does it mean to feel at home in a hospital?

"Have you packed your bag?" There are lists of things that the woman should take to the hospital to make her stay more comfortable. During labor, however, personal things are put away. The hospital garb is provided, which helps the woman to fit into the patient role. I think back on Paula's birth experience. She had planned ahead—freezing the meal to be served after the birth, letting her mother-in-law know the kind of tea she preferred—and had prepared her home for this event. She drank her tea from her own cup—a special cup made by a friend especially for her. It was a clay cup with the iron particles showing through the glaze—round and smooth, nice to hold. During her labor, this cup, filled with warm soothing tea or refreshing cool water, expressed the care and nourishment that Paula needed to be reminded of as she endured her trial. The cup tied her to her friends and to the support she needed during the pain. How different this cup is from the styrofoam cup often used to bring a woman nourishment during labor in the hospital!

Many women talk of wanting to control the birth process. They want to be in control of their own experiences. In fact, the focus of many childbirth classes is to teach women how to use breathing patterns and controlled relaxation, or to prepare written birth plans in order to maintain as much control as possible. And it was control that the birthing-room parents said they valued. Yet, one has to wonder what this focus on control is really about. Is it really control that is desired? To be able to go with labor and its pain, one has to lose control—to let the body do its work, to ride the wave of the pain. The fact that one cannot control the uterus any more than one can control one's heart means that the woman needs to abandon herself to the process (Nathanielsz 1992). Perhaps in order to gain control one has to lose it. A strange possibility. Yet, if women know they have control of their environment, they may be more free to abandon inner control and follow the "out of control-ness" of their laboring body. In such a supportive environment women would be able to pick up control again whenever they chose to (Morgan 1984). What is important is that women need to feel comfortable (as though they are at home), so that their need to express their pain through a change of position, having friends and family near, making noise, or receiving medication is supported. It may appear from this discussion that the home is the best place to birth a child; however, in many situations, the home may not be a good place at all.

Support During Pain

"I thought of the millions, literally billions of women who have experienced this pain, and if they could experience it, then I can too. That made me feel strong," remembers Anna. The knowledge that women share with other women has been lost in the replacement of midwives by doctors (primarily male) as birth attendants. This loss is being recognized. Women's challenge to regain control of the childbirth process is a recognition of the importance of sharing the bodily knowing of childbirth with other women, as a mother would. "After all, *I did it*! It was hard. It was long. I did rely on my instincts. I did rely on my friends. In a very real sense, we did it together. After my first child, I felt, and continue to feel, that I'd always have an affinity with other women, unnamed but real," says Paula. "I can't begin to envision the nightmare and horror of carrying on (in the pain) without being in an atmosphere of caring and loving people."

Support for women in labor pain must be there without the asking. They need support from partners and friends as well as from the experts. Support may take the form of back rubs, suggestions, sips of cool water, a cup of warm tea, a soothing touch, words of encouragement, the presence of a caring person, the quiet of the room, and an acknowledgment that what is happening is normal and expected. Women need to be reminded that the pain is there because pain is integral to the nature of birthing, not necessarily because something is wrong. While there needs to be direct verbal and physical support, there also needs to be recognition and respect for the privacy of the pain. As Paula remarks, "I especially appreciated everyone's silence while I rested on my side. I knew people were with me, there was never a doubt in my mind." Yet in this inwardness there is an attentiveness to the deep significance of the momentous quality of the pain. This is important pain, "a sacred fire." Laura Brown remembers, "I was annoyed when someone was making light conversation with my husband. I felt it was disturbing and irrelevant to what was happening to me." "It was an incredible sensation being totally into myself. I didn't have thoughts. I was really in tune with my body. I think it must be something in you that just happens. In meditation you can go so far but this was much, much different. In those last few hours there was no straying of the mind. I couldn't talk because I was on one plane and he [her husband] was on another. Mine was an inward focus" (Victoria LeClair). This deeply felt experience reaches to the core and Plessner has shown "Pain means being thrown back on ourselves" (Buytendijk 1961: 131). Pain demands women to muster up even more strength to survive, to live through it. But not alone. "I look at Marie and I see the terror of childbirth in her eyes. I feel it. I remember it. I know it can be survived. I tell her so" (Harrison 1982: 105).

In aiding the laboring woman, one must recognize her authority and the reality of pain and difficulty. One must encourage her to use her special capacities to deal with the pain as a creative action of nature and not as oppression (Kittay 1983: 124). For example, comments like "Perhaps you need a sedative" may lead to personal doubt and loss of confidence. Is it possible that the offer of medication to obliterate pain is sometimes accepted by a woman simply because it is the only support that is offered in the face of the overwhelming sensation of pain? The offer of medication confirms the fear that, yes indeed, she will not be able to stand it. This is not to say that a woman does not need the help of medication—but the offer of medication should not be the first or, indeed, the only support that is extended.

While recognizing the need for a supportive community during the painful birth experience, a woman may begin to grasp the reality of her aloneness. As she is pervaded by a deep sense of inwardness, she is compelled to acknowledge her selfhood, to be conscious of her own existence. Victoria comments, "I feel great for the process to have happened through my body, proud of realizing such stamina, strength, and determination." The woman learns about the strengths she has. She has climbed a mountain, reached a summit. She understands her own strengths and capabilities in a new way.

The Time of Pain

It's time! Her time has come! The baby is coming! The pains tell the time. As the pains begin, women feel excitement and apprehension. This is what they have been waiting for. This is it! Yet, what is known? Women may know the stages of labor, know the procedures to expect, know some things to do, and yet ask, "How will I handle it?" What will it *really* be like? Each time we know more about what to expect and do, but the mystery of *this* time is still present. Each time is its own time.

"It is a different kind of pain—like muscle cramps or extremely bad gas. It comes and goes—that is the reward, that it goes away," says Jane. Further exploration of the etymology of the word "birth" shows that "to bear children" is tied to the Old Norse root *bara* meaning wave, billow, or bore. A bore—a high and often dangerous wave caused by the surge of a flood tide upstream in a narrowing estuary or by colliding tidal currents—is a good image for labor. "This wave imagery is closely associated with the idea of rhythm. . . . With each wave of the sea the tide gradually flows farther in, bringing nearer the time when her baby will be in her arms" (Kitzinger 1979: 85). The contractions of birthing, like the colliding of the tidal currents, are most painful at the point when the baby moves down the "narrow estuary" of the birth canal. The description of birth as a series of waves tells us about the coming and going of the pain, the developing intensity, the climax, the release, and the moment of gathering resources for the next coming of the pain wave.

When women talk about the time of labor, they think of timing the contractions. "We started to time them, seven minutes, ten minutes, and then at about 10:30 they went to about four minutes, lasting about thirty or sixty seconds. It wasn't hard for me," says Christine. "When I first went into labor it was about midnight—about five minutes apart, these funny twinges" remembers Susan. The timing of the contractions gives helpful hints as to what is happening, for we know that the longer and stronger are the pains, the farther into labor the woman has progressed. Yet even this timing can be overdone, with pages of records of contractions, for after a point most women know the nature of their contractions. The more women are assisted to recognize their own body rhythm, the more they may be able to flow with its pain in the process of birthing their children. "It was as if the pain was all there was. It would never end. There would be no result. I would live it forever," says Paula. During labor there is no sense of growth and change, but the cessation of time. There is no intention, only the will to endure.

The Baby and the Mother

"And then I couldn't believe the sensation because it was . . . as soon as I saw him, it was as if everything was gone and it gets very blurry," says Susan. Victoria talks of her changing relationship: "I couldn't take my eyes off him. I cut the cord—cutting the cord, really making the break from the baby. One relationship dies and another relationship begins." Deliver, deliverance, the act of transferring to another. The pains are a literal expression of the narrow gateway leading to release in the expanse of life. The involvement changes from the self-as-world to the baby-as-world. As the body releases the baby, the pain is released. The attention is turned to the new life, the new being. "Something in me was released. I turned away from my somewhat egotistic involvement in my labor toward my child, and since that moment my love has grown . . . so much that it actually hurts sometimes" (Kitzinger 1977: 161). The pain is released, with the possibility of a new and different pain tied to the incredible and awesome awareness of a separate being. The woman who becomes mother vastly increases her capacity for pain and vulnerability.

With the pain of childbirth women become mothers. Can pain be transformed into something usable, asks Rich (1976: 151), "something which takes us beyond the limits of our experience itself—into a further grasp of the essentials of life and the possibilities within us?" What is it that is learned? "I think I have a right to feel good about myself. In a way, this birth is helping me to accept myself—both the limitations and the capabilities. Accepting myself is the other side of the coin of accepting the pain," says Paula. Anna remarks, "I would never have wanted it any other way. It gave me confidence and strength. I was able to deal with the pain, to confront and overcome. Now I know that I can deal with it, and that is useful in encountering other painful things." To have experienced birthing pain offers the possibilities of self-knowledge, knowledge of limitations and capabilities, of new life as a mother, and of a woman's place in the mysterious cycle of human life—birth, death, and rebirth. As women give birth to children, they, in a sense, birth themselves. They become mothers, like their own mothers, and as their daughters probably will after them. "There is that sisterhood. There is a knowing that you, as a mother, have gone through what I've gone through," observes Anna. Victoria also recognizes the tie to other mothers: "Rose was the only other mother there. I had something in common with her. I started to cry when she hugged me."

THE RESPONSIBILITY

The fragility of life is startling. The baby's first breath leaves us in awe at its tenuousness. To become a mother can feel like an overwhelming responsibility—a terrifying one—especially when something goes wrong. An incident sticks in my mind from when my son was small. He was younger than four, sick with a cold or flu, and his fever was rising. I felt his forehead, soothed his restlessness, wondered what to do. My hand moved to his pulse and a jolt went through me—his pulse was rapid and erratic, fitful, all over the place! What did this mean? Was something wrong with his heart? How did this happen? What can I do now? To become a mother involves responsibility for the birth and life of another person, the child.

Anna Gurley. Is this what having a kid is like?

Anna and Bill talk often about taking responsibility for the birth of their child. They have carefully considered their decision to have a home birth, weighing all the evidence for safety as well as what seems best for them. We talk together in their home four or five times, and both Anna and Bill discuss their decision for home birth many times. Bill says, "My sister, who was initially against the idea, is actually envious of us. She admires us for doing it, she thinks it takes courage. But we don't think it is taking courage, it is taking what it really is, the ultimate in responsibility, that responsibility if something goes wrong. In a hospital there is always someone to attach responsibility or blame to. But if it happens at home, we will have to be responsible." Anna agrees. "I have thought of the potential of . . . let's say the baby doesn't make it. If it is in the hospital everyone would say that the doctor tried his very best, and if it should happen at home, we are going to be seen as irresponsible, killers, and murderers. That is pretty drastic and I guess I am willing to live with that.

"I think we [society] deny death. For how many people is death a real thing? How many have seen a dead person? Or touched a dead person? We have dehumanized death, just as hospitals have dehumanized birth through interventions and goodness knows what else. I think that for us a birth at home is less of a risk than the hospital. People do not want to believe that it is safer at home because they want to put the responsibility into the hands of the doctor and the hospital. Of course, I will go to the hospital if I have to, but I really prefer not to."

Anna and Bill puzzle about why so many people who talk in a negative way about their hospital experiences with childbirth still go back to the same situation the next time. Anna states, "I think some of the negative experiences are because men are very protective, or else they doubt our capabilities and maybe that is why they are protective. I think it is all tied up in the man/woman relationship, with man trying to be superior to woman and maybe envious of woman's capability to have children. Doctors/obstetricians often want to take credit for the delivery."

"Is that true for you?" I ask Bill, "Do you feel that you would like to have the baby yourself?" Bill says he does not feel envious. He says, "I know that there is something going on there that I will never, never, know about. I think, sometimes I feel that there is a bond being established right now that I, as much as I would like to, can't be a part of. Because it is just not possible. But I like, by our closeness, to feel that I get a look. There is always going to be something dear and special about a mother and child relationship. No matter what qualities I bring to it, it is something I can't hope to penetrate. I think that is the protectiveness that a lot of men have toward women." But to this Anna reacts, "You see, I don't think that protectiveness is a valid, honest feeling for men to have, for the doctor to have, because, let's face it, women are built for the situation. The body takes care, the body does it all. We don't need episiotomies, we don't need enemas, we don't need to be shaved, the body takes care of it. One of the things you have to think about is if the child doesn't make it, is stillborn or . . . I think it would be better to be home. It is the best place to experience that, where you have your friends and your loved ones around with you. Birth and death are on a continuum, I think, and as hard as that would be, I'd prefer to be at home, and we have prepared for that."

"And then when she did come out, her face was quite blue. She was limp, had no reflexes, she didn't grimace or sneeze or do any of that kind of stuff. Her heart rate was good, but her respiration was irregular and slow, and her color was blue. She didn't make any noise." Anna is speaking about her newborn baby, whom she holds in her arms. Bill, Carol (her sister), Kate (Carol's eighteen-month-old daughter), and I are sitting in their home drinking coffee. Bill continues, "After she had the oxygen, she started breathing and sputtering and crying. Her Apgar score was only four at one minute. It was pretty scary. The midwife was very calm. She did what she had to do. But after it was all over, the midwife too was shaking." Anna, in a calm voice, describes what happened next, "Jena really recovered well, though. Within about two minutes she began to cry and that was just wonderful. We didn't even know whether she was a boy or girl at that point of time. She was on my tummy."

"It took a while to sort of get over that," says Bill. "I guess I thought that any breathing problems would be more a result of drugs in hospitals, so I was really taken aback by all this. And I thought, 'Oh, my gosh, is this what having a kid is like? Terror like this? Will she be okay? Will she be okay tomorrow? Will she be okay the day after?' "

Taking Responsibility

We may talk about taking responsibility for ourselves and for the child, as Anna did during pregnancy, but when there is an actual child in our lives, a child entrusted to us (and even the child as stranger) who is not breathing properly, has an erratic heartbeat, or is heard crying amidst the rubble of an earthquake, we are transformed by a sense of responsibility that subjects us to a certain terror that is not present in talk. We are shocked by our helplessness as we come face to face with the reality of illness, deformity, or death of the child we accepted in our life. What leads to a sense of responsibility that has such profound dimensions? Is this what having a child is like?

To have a healthy baby, the pregnant woman must be healthy. She is told by everyone—doctors, nurses, family, and friends—that she now must look after herself. As soon as she is pregnant, or even before, the woman is encouraged to eat right and to avoid alcohol, tobacco, drugs, and even coffee. She is encouraged to get enough sleep, enough exercise, and enough fresh air. She is warned against microwaves, computer monitors, X-rays, ultrasound, and too much exercise, and is even told "You shouldn't lift things over your head." Women are becoming more and more conscious of the association between environmental and substance toxins and fetal abnormalities. They are aware that their responsibility begins very early, even before they get pregnant. Pre-conception information encourages this early responsiveness on the part of women, as does public scrutiny—even threats of incarceration and labels on cigarette packages and alcohol bottles.

So women look after themselves and pay attention to their bodies in ways they did not before pregnancy. Some women may find it easier to quit smoking when there is "someone else" to think about. Yet, some may not. They may become more responsive, and responsible, once they are convinced that there is a baby present. When they feel the movement, hear the heartbeat, and see the kicks and rumbles across their stomachs, they begin to sense the reality of the baby. For some, ultrasound makes the baby's presence more real. "I had an ultrasound at eleven weeks. The baby was all there. Whole. It came real to me because of that. I didn't feel pregnant but it brought everything into focus," says Christine.

But "taking care" may not be enough. The increasing number of technological investigations, such as amniocentesis and ultrasound, is a constant reminder that, in spite of their care of themselves, women may bear a baby with congenital disease and handicaps, or develop high blood pressure, toxemia, or other diseases associated with pregnancy that could threaten their baby and themselves. Although Susan faithfully ate her veggies, as she says, she was still afraid that her body would let her down and her baby would not make it. Women also wonder about the possibility of a deformed child and worry about their ability to "deal with it—living with a child that has mental or physical problems on a day-to-day basis," as Anna puts it. The problem of risk, however, is more complex. Some women have more risk than others and—sometimes the technology itself is a risk.

As women get closer to the time of birth, they begin to feel their responsibility to get things—like the baby's clothes and the baby's room—ready. They also get ready for their own labor experience. They pack their bag, and in their bag they may have a birth plan that they have worked out with the midwife or doctor. They have chosen the person, usually the child's father or a close woman friend, who will be with them. They are ready. But when Anna talks of taking the responsibility for the birth, she describes how she sterilized the towels and sheets, how she purchased the protective sheet for the bed, and even, early on, how she found a place to live that would accommodate the home birth. She says, "It was almost a ritual to sterilize the towels and things. It was good to do that because to a certain extent you're overwhelmed by the responsibility. I don't think I would encounter that if all I did was to pack a bag and go to the door of the hospital. It is a different kind of preparation." The actual physical preparation (sterilizing the towels and purchasing the pads) helps Anna to prepare to take the responsibility for giving birth.

Anna is the only mother in this study who talks about the possibility of the death of her child during labor and delivery. Of course, this is understandable since she chose to birth her child outside the bounds of approved practice. Thus she is open to all the "what if" questions that hospital care is presumed to deflect. Anna worries about the censorship she would feel if something happened to the baby, but then she says, "I think that for us a birth at home is less of a risk than the hospital. I think people do not want to believe that it is safer at home because they want to put the responsibility into the hands of the doctor and the hospital." For Anna having the baby at home and getting things ready for the birth helps her to move to motherhood through accepting responsibility for herself and her child in a way that she could not if she planned to go to a hospital.

Women are ready when the time comes. The frequent trips to the bathroom, the difficulty in moving around and in finding a comfortable position for sleep, the need to eat small, more frequent meals, all of these problems make each woman ready. But what does it mean to be ready? While Susan McLaren thinks it is time for the birth, that her body is ready, she wonders about her readiness in another sense. "Gee, am I ready for this? I am going to be thirty-two, I'd better be ready. I think it's like starting any new job, you know. I didn't feel like a teacher until I started doing it."

Embodied Responsibility

Women are made ready by experiencing the responsibility through their bodies. Many are aware of their pregnancy before they "know for sure" from a pregnancy test or the doctor's examination. Christine was so sure that, in spite of the fact that the pregnancy test was negative, she said to her doctor, "Treat me as if I am, because I am." Katherine, also, was sure, so she didn't need to purchase the pregnancy kit that contains two tests. One would do. Susan, on the other hand, had lost faith in her body, was fed up with her body not doing things right, so she did not consider her very sore breasts—so uncomfortable that she had a hard time walking up and down stairs—as a possible sign of pregnancy. Women depend on the doctor's examination for confirmation. Yet, dependency on the pregnancy test, the doctor's examination, and other recent technological devices, such as ultrasound, may devalue their own body knowledge.

A pregnant woman feels the movements of the baby and the contractions of her uterus with an immediacy and certainty that no one else can share; but with the increasing use of techniques and machines such as ultrasound and fetal monitoring, her experiential knowledge is reduced in value, replaced by what is seen as more reliable knowledge. Therefore it is easy for a woman to lose touch with or doubt her own experience, and to accept objective knowledge as more correct and therefore valuable.

Menstruation is one of the first signs that remind women, and society, that complete control of female bodies is not possible. Perhaps this is why it is viewed so negatively by a society that, above all else, venerates control. This desire to control is so entrenched that even menstruation is denigrated in the effort to control it. In pregnancy, the woman shares her body with the growing child, an experience characterized by fatigue, weight gain, nausea, flatulence, shortness of breath, vulnerability, and clumsiness that can be only partially controlled. In fact, these uncomfortable bodily experiences are a part of a healthy pregnant woman's life. Labor is structured into stages in an effort to manage and predict, but each woman's labor has its own rhythm, pattern, and progression that left alone passes in its own time. The baby, too, with a rhythm all its own, demands that time move with its pace ("fetal time," as it is called by Rapp 1984: 314). The effort to control, for example to control death, especially the death of a baby, creates the dilemmas that now confront us, like the "right to die," which might be equally important as to "live at all costs" (Colen 1986; McDermott 1986). The death of a baby is beyond our comprehension, it seems—we must do everything (even apprehend) the child if there is the slightest chance of death.

Humility, the virtue needed to take on a world beyond our control, "emerges from maternal practices and accepts not only the reality of damage and death, but also the actuality of the independent and uncontrollable life of nature" (Ruddick 1983: 217). Humility, when confused with self-effacement (humility's degenerative form), is a negative image that secular society abhors. Nevertheless, true humility, developed in the face of life's uncontrollable situations, is a quality to be treasured. Faith in women's bodies gives power, not power "over" but power to "go with," to move within the forces of body knowledge. Such faith gives women the confidence needed to take charge of their own environments and allows them to live autonomously, to be self-reliant, and to make individual choices in line with their own sense of values. Women who mother are transformed by the recognition that complete control of life, as the control of death, is an illusion.

Obstetrical science does not easily place itself in a humble relationship to the reality of the puzzle of life, which includes death and other aspects that are out of human control (Young 1987). In the effort to control and manage life (and death) there is the potential for usurping women's need to develop the sense of responsibility that giving birth entails. Brenda

Watson's husband's wish for a cesarean birth gives a clue to the problem that is faced by women. Brenda says, "Now he wants me to have a cesarean so he can watch them take it out from the other side. He says it is more humane, like he didn't like to have the woman suffer." While it is important to control suffering, one should also consider that the challenge faced by women in childbirth, in the experience of labor, may have a value that comes with accepting responsibility.

For women who mother, not only is there tension between the commitment to the child and to oneself, but there is another reason for ambivalence. Once a child comes into one's life there is always a fear of losing the child. The woman giving birth is the icon of the birth-death cycle, of the finiteness of the human condition. We are born to live and to die. Although the modern agenda is to develop knowledge that will prevent disability and death, loss and death are real possibilities. Ultimately, the life and death of the child are beyond human control.

In the effort to control nature for the perfect baby, what may be bypassed is the quality of life, that is, the whole picture. The whole picture includes the child and the mother. Birth is not just for the child or just for the mother. It is a relational activity. The mother's realization and acknowledgment of the strength and power of her reproductive body is realized in her ability to birth her own child. Pregnancy and birth can be likened to the progression and intensity of sexual pleasure in intercourse. What happens when women miss the orgasm, the release that leads to satisfaction and contentment?

The Space of Responsibility

Today much discussion about childbirth focuses on the place of birth. Most women and medical personnel agree that the hospital is the preferred location, primarily because of the proximity to lifesaving expertise and machines. Women generally feel they are taking responsible action by following this trend. They do not wish to take a chance. Yet some women are beginning to realize that the hospital environment may not be the most favorable place for this intimate event to take place. Both Anna Gurley and Katherine Lang chose to deliver their babies at home. Anna and Katherine felt that a home birth offered the opportunity for them to act on their own good judgment and authority rather than under the authority of others, such as the doctor and hospital staff. The issue is not safety: both women were making choices based on the literature that states that with a normal birth, the home is as safe, or even safer, than a hospital (Mehl, Peterson, Whitt, and Hawes 1977; Hoff and Schneiderman 1985). For these women, proximity to emergency care was an important consideration.

All the women spoke of childbirth as a normal, natural event. Up until the time of the birth all took responsibility for themselves—they watched their nutrition, exercised, went for their regular checkups, and took prenatal classes. Yet, like most women, Brenda, Christine, Jane, and Susan chose a place of birth in which they would be safe in the hands of others. Our present Canadian healthcare environment does not provide adequate medical support proximate to the home (e.g. emergency medical services such as flying medical squads), so hospital care is the most appropriate choice for many women. What does choosing a place of birth have to do with responsibility? Katherine hints at this question as she describes her move from home to hospital during labor. "When I went into hospital things really changed for me in the sense that all of a sudden there were a lot of things done to me. I was a patient. It was a real change—a turning point. From then on things were really out of my hands."

When I visited Brenda in the hospital the day after the birth, I was reminded of the fact that, although I was visiting her, both of us were visitors in the hospital. The rituals that occur in the hospital environment demonstrate how responsibility shifts from the personal authority of the woman to the authority and responsibility of the hospital staff and hospital routine (Kelpin and Martel 1984). Etymologically, "hospital" is a doublet of "hotel," and both words presuppose that someone enters into a "hospitable" place, as a guest or a hostess. The hospital, as we know it, is the place where sick people enter in order to be restored to health or to die. "You know what struck me," Christine says hesitantly, "when you go through admitting, they ask your name, number, and so on. Don't you know I'm in labor! I wanted to say. It was so routine to them, so boring for them, just routine business." The exciting reality of labor and the formal routine of entering the hospital were at odds.

Next, Christine was taken up to the ward. She says, "They did a lot to me. I can't tell you a lot of the things that happened between arrival and getting into bed. It's vague." Activity was all around her but she just wanted to relax. Christine's words display the gap between what she wanted to experience, that is, the relaxing of her body, and what was seen as necessary for her admission to the hospital. Her concentration was focused inward, while the admission procedures forced her attention outward. The ward is a world of anonymous people, nurses whose names and faces she could not remember. They were introduced to her but she could not remember who they were. As her attention was turned inward, the people around her remained faceless and her surroundings remained vague. Attired according to the status of a patient, Christine entered further into the world of medicine, characterized by passivity and obedience. Her gratefulness at being in a quiet room alone with her husband shows Christine's underlying desire for autonomy or independence in an environment that supports her need for relaxation and inward attention.

Does the use of a birthing room change this gradual assimilation into the hospital environment and the "patienthood" that Christine experienced?

The staff at the hospital where Susan gave birth left her and her husband, Paul, alone much of the time during labor, after checking the fetal heart with the stethoscope. Susan's main concern during labor was that she did not make too much noise. She wanted to fit in without a fuss. "By the time you fit yourself around the hospital's schedule—breakfast at a certain time, and then exercises, and then the baby is brought in to be bathed and fed—there is not much time left."

Jane arrived at the hospital about two hours before Lisa's birth and was pleased that the birthing room was available. "It was great," she says, "it was carpeted and there was music playing, with a little television beside the bed, and a telephone near." She was put on the fetal monitor right away, and once her membranes had been ruptured by the resident doctor, the external apparatus was replaced with internal electrodes. Jane thought the membranes were ruptured because they were so busy they needed the room and "didn't want me to take any more time than I had to." The nurses and doctors were helpful, giving directions to guide the birth. Jane remembers, "All of a sudden, in the middle of a contraction, I had to push. They said, 'Don't push, don't push.' I could breathe through those all right." The doctor was not there, so a resident came, scrubbed, gowned, and kept saying to her, "Don't push, don't push." Then her doctor arrived and said, "Breathe, breathe," until he was ready. "By the time I was allowed to push," says Jane, "I was really ready to push. Jim was really my saving grace, as he kept saying, 'Don't push, breathe.' He kept me on track. Even then, when I got pushing, they wanted me to stop so they could do an episiotomy. That was really tough." Jane talks about her amazement at seeing her tiny baby with a head that looked so big. The doctor held her up, before they cut the cord, and said to Jane, "Look, don't touch, but look at her."

Jim was Jane's saving grace, keeping her on track according to the directions and wishes of the doctors and nursing staff. Jane was only allowed to push when they were ready. For most of her labor Jane was at home, where it had progressed normally as she followed the rhythm of her laboring body in a supportive environment with her husband and parents. When she went to the hospital and moved toward birth, she was told what to do so that the staff and their procedures could be accommodated—waiting for the doctor, the scrubbing, the dressing, the episiotomy. Now she needed to be "kept on track," to look but not touch, and to be "saved" by others. Has the birthing room really enabled women to gain access to the lifesaving capabilities of medical science without depriving them of their own life-giving prerogatives? In whose hands is birth?

When I visited Anna the day after the birth of Jena, the situation was very different. Anna and Jena, along with Anna's sister Carol and her two-year-old daughter, Nicky, were together in their living room. Nicky held the baby. Anna served me coffee. A short time later Bill arrived with a big box of diapers. They were at home. I was the guest. By virtue of it being their home, their space, they were in control. By being in control of their space, they were able to allow the birth process to proceed in its own time. Anna felt she was in control most of the time during her labor (although she nearly "lost it" in transition). Yet during the labor itself one expects to lose control—the contractions of the uterus, the pain, the intensity take over—and by going with it, in a sense by losing control, one gains control. "The midwives were incredible," says Bill, "they were so unobtrusive. They didn't do a lot during labor, they were so patient. It was wonderful to have them here to check the fetal heart, but because we were managing, they stayed in the background." Bill goes on to say, "We did it ourselves," which is what I think women want when they say they want control. They want to do it themselves, to be self-reliant without losing the support of others.

In the hospital it is easy for the doctors, the nurses, and others to take responsibility: it is their space. At home, although the midwives are present, the responsibility falls on the mother (or parents): it is their space. No matter how the hospital rooms are "dolled up" (Anna's term) with the cozy quilt, the rocking chair, and the telephone, the homelike hospital is still a strange place, a foreign space—"might as well have the green walls and the harsh lights," says Anna. A foreign space, by the very fact that it is not home, creates a problem of control, of "whose hands it is in." Yet again, perhaps it is not control at all that is desired, rather self-reliance—the difference is a tricky one. Even in the birthing room there is a need for staff to relinquish control, so that a woman can be free to follow the intuitive knowledge embodied in her birthing body, to "go with" rather than to "manage" the birthing process. "For a woman to attain autonomy she need not renounce her biological capacities, but gain control over them" (Kittay 1983: 133). In gaining control she has the opportunity to relinquish her control to the autonomy of her own birth-giving body and its process. Hospital environments can be made to be home away from home not only with changed decor, but also with a philosophy that puts women at the center. It is the woman who gives birth, within the arms of a caring partner and with the assistance and support of knowledgeable people. Nothing is taken away from her own process, and as she births the child she can begin to respond to that child, nourishing the child by offering the breast and moving toward the responsibility of mothering.

Responsible Relationships

One of the first things a woman does when she finds herself pregnant is to choose a doctor or midwife. The process of shopping around for someone who will support a woman's needs, desires, and priorities is now encouraged by childbirth educators and consumer advocates. "The choice of care giver and a place of birth determine, to a great extent, the kind of birth experience you will have" (Simkin, Whalley and Keppler 1984: 5). Some doctors, according to Anna, want to take credit for the birth. She and Bill, her husband, feel that their choice of doctor and midwife helps them to take their own responsibility for the pregnancy, the birth, and the child. Recall Anna's comment about the chance of the death of their child—they will be seen "as irresponsible, as killers, and murderers." Pretty strong words. They would be responsible. It is different for Brenda. She says, "Whatever will be, will be." Everything was left to her doctor's discretion. For many years pregnant women have been used to accepting the idea that the obstetrician should take over the guardianship of the woman for twelve months. A 1961 obstetrics text states that the physician "supervises food intake, regulates activities, answers questions, clarifies puzzlements, and advises on handling the baby when it comes and generally charts her activities during the twenty-four hours of the day" (Seiden 1978: 92). Many women are not willing to accept such patronizing anymore, but sometimes find it hard to achieve a healthy balance of cooperation with those to whom they go for care.

There was often talk about the sex of the baby. Will the baby be a boy or a girl? Of course, it does not really matter. Or does it? Women realize that there is a responsibility to society to raise an acceptable child (Ruddick 1983). What kind of girl or boy is acceptable to present society? Christine, pregnant with her second child, says that this time "we would really like a baby girl. Yet I kind of think, you know what?" speaking very quietly, " kind of think I don't know if I want a girl, just because I don't know if I want her to face this world as a woman. I still think that men have an easier time. I would want my little girl to just go for it, like I think I have, and then I get quite concerned about the kinds of things she is going to have to go through or over—get over—to be a person in this world. I have ambivalent feelings about it. It would be fine, but . . . " Christine thinks it would be easier to raise a boy, because you could be direct and tell him what the world is like. With a girl there would be more of a dilemma. "My little girl would learn from me, but I'd have to tell her, we do this here but in the real world [that] will happen. I wonder if I could prepare my girl child for the world as well as I could my boy child." To have a son or a daughter does not seem to be a problem for most parents as they say, "it doesn't matter, as long as the baby is healthy." Yet they want a balanced family, and after one or two daughters they may wish for at least one son. The technology is available to create gender imbalances through the deliberate choice of the sex of the child. Technology (particularly amniocentesis and ultrasound) brings the age-old patriarchal dream of selecting the child of the right sex into the real world. It happens! Recognition of the value of women, of girl children, and their contribution to society must occur in the public arena if the hesitations that Christine and others speak about are to be avoided. In a community that treasures girls and boys for their unique contributions, parents would not choose a boy over a girl or a girl over a boy, but would welcome every child, and help each of them grow to become a valued member of the community.

Many people who witness the birth of a child experience awe and wonder. They sense the connectedness of life, of mother and child, of mother and father, of mother and midwife or doctor, even the ultimate connectedness of all humanity, since it is how we all begin our lives. Giving birth to a child is at the same time mysterious and knowable, mundane and sacred, commonplace and unique; it gives life and it leads to death. These characteristics are not opposites, or polarities, they are one and the same thing.

In the next chapter I discuss women's experience of adoption, which includes the experience of both the birth mother and the adopting mother. I take up again the themes of the decision, the presence of baby, the pain of mothering, and the responsibility to show how mothers involved in adoption experience these themes. With adoption the notion of belonging comes out in full color—how children belong and how mothers belong. The difference between ownership and belonging is emphasized.

NOTE

Earlier versions of this chapter were written as part of doctoral research completed in 1986 and published in 1989 in a book entitled *Woman to Mother: A Transformation*. Granby, Mass.: Bergin & Garvey Publishers.

3

Adoption's Two Mothers

> We don't communally understand why we want children. I think that might be true for people who just have children as much as for people who want them but can't have them. People who have wanted children for a long time are inclined to sit down and think about it. I'm sure that if I had had a child at twenty-eight I would have never thought about it. At that age it is something that just happened to you—in the course of your life. (Joan Bell, 46 years)

Where does the desire for children come from? Is it innate in our bodies? Is it culturally expected? Is it just assumed to happen in the course of a life? Understanding the reasons and the desire to have children is not straightforward. The desire for a child is experienced differently by different women. This chapter focuses on the experience of women who choose to adopt a child and women who choose to place their child for adoption. The women who talked to me about adoption and placement are unique. They are not a sample of all women; rather, they are a particular group, many of whom used the services of one private adoption agency to facilitate the transfer of responsibility of a child from one woman to another. The agency works with birth mothers (and sometimes with birth fathers) who need to place and with couples (usually) who wish to adopt. My focus is on the experiences of the women, both the birth mothers and the adopting mothers.

When one explores adoption from the point of view of experience, one must consider the experience of both the birth mothers and the adopting mothers at the same time—for one cannot exist without the other. Through adoption, the giving mothers (birth mothers, placing mothers) and receiving mothers (adopting mothers) launch a never ending connection. The voices of the women in this chapter are based on conversations with adopting and placing mothers that took place during an intense period in their lives. I met with the birth mothers one to three times during their experience of late pregnancy and after the child was born and placed. I met with the adopting mothers one to four times from their experience of application to a period following receiving the child. I asked both birth mothers and adopting mothers to describe (in whatever way they wished) what the experience of adoption was like for them.

OPEN ADOPTION

The women in this study have primarily experienced open adoption. In the open adoption arrangement there is a meeting of the two women, the two mothers. The contact between them over the subsequent years varies from frequent personal contact to occasional letters spaced at agreed-upon intervals. The women know who each other are, have met and talked together, and have made some kind of an agreement about the manner and extent of the contact between the birth mother and the adopted child.

Connie Hancock knew that for her to have a child she would need to adopt. She chose to use the services of an agency that offers open adoptions. When I first spoke with Connie, she was ready to adopt. In fact, she says, she was ready yesterday.

Connie Hancock. Ready yesterday

"Vulnerable," "full of terror," "fearful," "awkward" are the descriptive words that Connie used when she talks of the adopting process. Connie discovered at seventeen that she would never carry or give birth to a child. She did not have a uterus; she had ovaries, but no uterus. "I was absolutely devastated. I'm sure I was in a daze—probably for a couple of years. Just couldn't believe it. I knew that adoption was the only way that we would have a child. All my friends have children now. And I'm always on the outside kind of looking in. I *really* want to be a mother. It has been four years since we were married and we were missing out. I want to have a family! Like, it's just so lonely."

Connie had chosen to work with small babies and had seen some difficult situations of adoption. She knew that adoption was not a bed of roses, yet she still wanted to go for it. She felt at the mercy of others throughout the adoption process: through the home study, being chosen, meeting the birth mother and her family, at the birth, in the hospital, during the ten-day waiting period and the legal recognition that the child was her own. At all these times she was dependent on other people's assessment, needs, procedures, attitudes. She remarks, "The home study that we had was very intimidating, *very* intimidating. Because you really feel like you're at their mercy. You feel, you wouldn't want to say the wrong thing. After our first little bit of hesitation—a bit panic stricken, terror really—we just started talking and it just started flowing. It really was because you're worried that, you know, well you're being evaluated the whole time and maybe you might say something that you don't really mean to say and she might take it the wrong way. And then life would pass us by.

"The social worker came out twice (for a three or four hour session both times), and will come again, in a year, if there hasn't been a placement. If there is a placement, she will do a postadoption report. The files are presented [to the birth mothers] in chronological order. So those that have been waiting longer have their files shown first—unless you have something that a birth mother specifically wants, for example, your religion, or, I don't know, something that they know that only you would serve, then your file would be pushed up.

"Actually I feel a lot more relaxed about it now than before we made the decision to adopt. In fact I remember we were away at Christmastime, and I just wasn't myself. When we came home, we made the decision. And I was happy then. Maybe there will be a positive outcome to all of this. "I think about what I would do when we get a phone call. About how quickly things have to move. You don't have nine months of anticipation of that date. Like we're sort of . . . your gestation period could be two months or it could be a year. I suppose I haven't really put a whole lot of thought into it other than knowing what I have to get and what I have to get quickly. I'd be ready tomorrow. I was ready yesterday!"

Open adoption is an arrangement facilitated through licensed private agencies, lawyers, or other professionals. The birth mother (sometimes the birth father) and the adopting parents apply to the agency and receive education, counseling, and assistance throughout the process, including the legalization of the adoption. The procedures may vary in different jurisdiction, but generally include the following stages:

a. attendance at an information session in which the process is described

b. home study of the adoptive parents by a social worker

c. contributions to a file by adopting parents (the "Dear Birth Mother" letter, references from family and friends, etc.)

d. completed adopters' file is shown to birth mothers

e. birth mother selects one or more couples as potential parents

f. adopting parents and birth mother (sometimes father) meet to discuss issues like ongoing contact

g. birth mother is counseled and supported before and after the birth and placement

h. birth mother signs consent form and baby goes home with the adopting parents

i. ten-day period where birth mother can legally change her mind

j. court appearance at about six months to legalize adoption

Open adoption is not an easy solution to the human experience of having an unplanned pregnancy, nor a cure for infertility for women who want a child. There are no easy solutions to the human dilemmas of having a child come too soon, or finding that a child does not come at all. Those who promote open adoption agree that severing all ties between birth and adoptive families affronts the best interests of everyone because in everyday reality, birth mothers and their children are inextricably connected—emotionally, medically, physically, and spiritually.

Adoption is established to benefit the child, that is, for children to have safe, nurturing homes in which to grow and parents who will provide that unconditional love and attention every child needs. Yet adoption, as experienced, must consider how a woman moves to take on the reality of being mother to a child she has not given birth to, and how a woman experiences placing the child born to her in someone else's care. Giving and receiving a child is not like giving and receiving any other gift—the child as gift involves matters of the heart and the soul, the body and the mind.

Adoption, as a way of becoming a mother, is sometimes said to be second best, an idea that derives from the notion that "ideally all children should be with their families of birth" (Ward 1993). Yet the women in this research, women who became mothers through adoption, say it is not second best, it is just *different*.

I think it is hard really facing the fact that you are not going to have a child yourself. It is hard. I didn't want to say, let's pretend it is the same: This is something different. It is valuable in its own way but it is different. (Joan Bell)

It has taken five years. At first it was completely foreign, and although we registered with Social Services [for adoption], it was a safety net for me. It was sort of like, "Well, I've taken care of that. Now God will let me get pregnant." It didn't happen and it was about two years of denial, and anger, and frustration with my whole system: no medical reason why I couldn't get pregnant, nothing wrong with my husband. Now, it is not important to either one of us that it come from your blood—when we got through that, we decided to proceed quickly with private adoption. [But] you have to be completely honest with yourself. If you go into it thinking that it is not different than having a child naturally, you're going to lose. It is completely different. The child is the same, the process is not even close—but it is not second best. (Jennifer Black)

Perhaps these women resist the judgment that "second best" implies, or perhaps, once women come to know that adoption is the only way for them to become mothers, adoption becomes, for them, the very best. For many women it may be the second choice, but not second best.

Open adoption places the difference directly in front of those involved, the mother and the child, the father, the grandparents—everyone. The reality of difference is that a birth mother is not a childless woman, but a mother who lives with an absent child (Connolly 1987), and an adopting mother is a woman who for many years, often too many years, has lived the life of a childless mother, a woman with a child on her mind. With open adoption there is frank acknowledgment that adoption is a different way to become a parent. Open adoption acknowledges the explicit reality of two mothers and exposes the myth that the adoptive family is a traditional family of one father and one mother, with children born to them. Open adoption, with its two mothers, two fathers, two families, results in a family constellation for which there is little social precedence. The move to openness can serve the best interests of all, the child, the birth mother, and the adopting parents. In many communities, such as Alberta, Canada, nowadays there is a trend toward more open adoptions, with different degrees of openness depending on the agency, the community, and the parents involved.

GIVING AND RECEIVING A CHILD

The idea of giving comes easily to our minds when we think of mothers staying up all night with a sick infant, or half the night waiting for a tardy teenager. Mothers are givers. And mothers are receivers too—giving and receiving love. But becoming a mother through adoption moves the idea of giving and receiving to a different plane, a plane that has stakes of enormous magnitude. With adoption it is not just giving and receiving for the sake of the child—it is the child who is given and received. With adoption, the giving and the receiving of the child as a gift have a string attached, a strong and elastic string that lasts a lifetime.

Often parents feel that a child is a gift—perhaps a gift to each other, or life's gift, or as gift of the Creator. Child as gift is an understandable notion. How else can one fathom the awe that we experience while holding a baby—that soft, warm, helpless, and trusting little being? The newborn baby exemplifies trust—trust that someone will feed, shelter, and care for him or her. In my own birth family, the belief that a child is a gift is made explicit. Each of us children has one name meaning "gift of God"—Daniel, Matthew, Dorothy, Theodore, Nathaniel, and, me, Theodora. Charlotte, too, talks about her adopted child, Betsy, as a gift—a precious spiritual gift. She describes holding Betsy, especially in those quiet early hours of the morning, as a profoundly religious experience. The birth mother is often thought to give the child as gift, a gift that makes adoptive mothers question, "How do you begin to say thank you?" Maybe that is why some parents can only really thank life, or fate, or God. This chapter is about the gift of a child. It is about how women experience the giving and the receiving of this precious and awesome gift.

The Birth Mother As Giver

When a woman comes to the point of adopting a child she often feels desperate for a child. She wants to be the receiver. She wants a birth mother to choose her as mother and to give her a child, even though at this time in her life it is hard for her to fathom giving a child of her own to anyone. But still, she knows that a child is a gift that is never really given away, for although the legal documents have parenting responsibilities transferred from birth to adopting mother, the birth bond is never dissolved. The umbilical cord, that physical cord cut at birth, is never truly severed, and in the back of everyone's mind there is that other person, be it birth mother or birth child. True, the thought of the other person may be submerged for years, but often, at some time in the lives of birth mothers and their birth children, that original connection pulls mother and child together again. A delightful example of desire for this reunion was recently published on the front page of a local newspaper (Staples 1995). Colleen Ransom (birth mother) and her daughter Jodi Vincent found each other through advertisements in the classified section printed next to each other on the same day—the day Jodi turned eighteen.

While the life-giving umbilical cord withers and drops off, the navel remains as an everlasting symbol of the bodily connection between mother and child, the bodily reminder of the presence, the touch, the pain, the emotion, the movement of the child carried beneath the birth mother's heart, as "part of you, part of your body, your flesh, your blood" (Cathy Bishop, a fifteen-year-old placing mother). This bodily experience of mother with child—*mamatoto*, Swahili for mother and child (Dunham et al. 1991), or *musukolome*, Kuranko for mother with child (Ross 1985)—is distinctive and unique, different from abstract notions of bloodlines, genetic links, or generational names. The birth mother's body is the child's first home, and is remembered, *in the body*, by both.

The notion of giving a child to someone else is hard to describe—what is being given, what is the gift? We hear the difficulty in the words used. For many years birth mothers were said to "relinquish" or "surrender" their babies for adoption. Now, birth mothers are encouraged to "place" their child. The idea of placing a child for adoption shows strong, definitive action. It signifies self-determination, independent thinking, rational decision-making, responsible action, and lack of coercion. It supports the idea of doing what is best for child and mother. It rings clearly of a generous, thoughtful gift, that of giving the child the best possibility in life, making someone else happy, doing something good for another, and/or doing the right thing. The placing mothers say:

I don't want my child to want for anything. I want him to have what he needs when he needs it. I just want more for my kid than what I was raised with, which was a single parent home and a lot of the times we didn't have a lot of food and stuff. We lacked for a lot when I was younger. So I don't want that for my child. (Lorrie Newton)

I just keep saying to myself that it's better off for the baby—and me. I want the best for him. It's hard to know you're giving away your child to someone. They'll not really know you. They'll be calling somebody else "Mum." (Mary Sebastian)

With Mary we begin to hear the anguish, the sorrow, the weeping that are juxtaposed to the seemingly clearheaded decision-making of these birth mothers. They say:

I'm really scared that I'm not going to be able to give it up. But I know it's the best thing for the baby right now, so I just keep telling myself, "Do the right thing. Do the right thing. Don't be selfish," you know. 'Cause it's my heart that'll be taking over. As soon as I see the baby. (Lorrie Newton)

I didn't have a choice. Because I couldn't keep my baby. I knew that for sure. Because it's just not a life I want when I have a baby. It wouldn't be a good life for a baby. I'm not ready. (Terry Lee)

These placing mothers give the child to the image of the right thing, the good mother, the good home, for all the good reasons; and they give up too, that is, they surrender or relinquish the child for exactly the same reasons. So while it seems that these mothers make rational and independent decisions, it may be really that they feel they have no other choice: Field (1992) reports that sixty percent of birth mothers feel they have little or no choice. They give up their baby to their own, and society's, ideal of the Good Mother. In this giving up we begin to hear the expectation of altruism of the birth mother: giving the good life so a child "does not want for anything" (Raymond 1990). In the accolades given to birth mothers who place—referred to as heroines or courageous souls—is there not a subtle coercion? After all, it is often thought that adoption is best for the child (for many good reasons), and that birth mothers who place their babies rather than keeping them have nothing to give the children themselves. Instead of giving of themselves to their child in active mothering, they give themselves and their child to the possibility of a good life, a better life than they had or than they think they can give. The women's stories show the reality of the gift they give in giving their child. The stories show how birth mothers give themselves in giving their babies for adoption.

Adopting mothers are the receivers of the gift of the child and worry how they can appropriately say "thank you" in a way that reflects the magnitude of the gift. Some think that having the birth mother share in the naming of the child is one way to express thanks. Giving the birth mother the right amount of contact with her child during the first year is also thought to be a way to ease the birth mother's sadness and guilt for having given up her child. For some adopting mothers, like Charlotte, receiving the child also takes time, time to feel entitled to say *my* baby rather than just *the* baby. To be called mother, to actually hold her child, after so many disappointments was an incredibly emotional time for Charlotte. Receiving the child is an act that moves woman to mother, a movement required for her to become the child's mother.

The Adoptive Mother As Chosen

With open adoption, it is not the child that is chosen, it is the mother. Although we often talk of the chosen child, with open adoption the reality of being a chosen mother is given stepwise precision. Of course, the adopting mother chooses to adopt, so the idea of the chosen child, that of "I wasn't expected, I was selected," has playful attractiveness. The adopting mother's decision to bring a child into her life is often more carefully weighed and deliberated than it is for many mothers. Women who adopt say that one of the hardest parts of adoption is "being at the mercy of others" and having such a major life event "out of your hands." Choice, with its power, is in the hands of the birth mother. Thus, in open adoption the adoptive mother is not chosen by God, nor by the courts, nor by the child, but, initially and ultimately, by the birth mother. Of course, some adoptive parents may state, like David and Faye Tearoe did when they heard the decision of the court to award custody of the baby to them, "God's hand was moved by our prayers" (Tanner 1993). Nevertheless, the initial move to give the child is made by the birth mother, who may later change her mind.

Prior to the choice by the birth mother, the adopting parents are examined and declared fit to be parents by society's representatives: the adoption agency, the social worker, the friends and family who send supporting letters, and the rules and regulations of the adoption process. The "Dear Birth Mother" letter written by the adopting parents is of utmost importance, requiring careful pondering on the part of the prospective adopting couple. It may be begun by her, then worked on by him, then revised and redone, in the effort to get it just right. Here the adopting parents outline why they would be good parents, hoping to say what the birth mother wants to hear, or as Lois Reynolds (an adoptive mother) says, "to show her that you can be what she wants you to be." The adopting mother wants to show herself as a good mother without actually saying so, because, continues Lois, "you can't brag about yourself or blow your own horn. It's hard to explain to someone how much you want children and how much everyone thinks you'd be a good parent." The adopting mother wants to show her happiness, the security of her life and marriage, her friendliness, her openness. In the letter she and her partner want to show the birth mother that as parents they are young enough, old enough, financially secure enough, down-to-earth enough, liberal enough, conservative enough, religious enough, committed enough, appreciative enough, and strong enough. The sturdy foundation of the white picket fence must be built. In the days or weeks it takes to write the letter to the birth mother, the adopting mother thinks about the qualities of the Good Mother, those perfect mothers, perfect parents who provide a good, safe, and secure home for the child. The adopting mother wants to be chosen, in fact, is desperate to be chosen. She wants to pass the test, a test she cannot study for, a test that most mothers do not have to even think about.

Desperation is sensed in the waiting and the anticipation: "Did the phone ring?" "Was the file shown?" "For sure by this time next year . . ." "I'm trying not to make it the center of my life." Nel Henry is not patient. She is anxious. "I am aching to have a child. I think we're up to probably twenty times [that our file has been shown] and we've never been chosen. We seem to live the lifestyle of a couple waiting to have a family. We often talk about that—maybe we should sell our middle-class lifestyle and become free-spirited, independent kind of people. Maybe we should live in a condo and travel six months of the year. But we don't. We fit into a more parental-type lifestyle." Her despairing "Yet, why is it taking so long? *Why is it taking so long?*" is heart-wrenching. Lois, too, worries about the reality of not being chosen, "Some think about the poor child who doesn't have a parent. Well, there are about a *thousand* parents waiting. Not like it used to be—*this poor little orphan.* What if you said the wrong thing? Or how would you feel if you knew she had picked you and then she met you and changed her mind? That would freak me out."

Needing to be chosen means being open to the possibility of rejection. And to be rejected as a parent is a terrible blow. "It is very frustrating," says Jennifer Black, "What is it about our file that is turning these people off? Is there anything we could do to fix it?" According to Karin Perry, "If you are rejected as a possible parent of a child, you are being rejected at a pretty fundamental aspect of being a human being." The adopting mothers lay their whole lives on the line, so to speak. The pages of the home study documents tell of attitudes, beliefs, and relationships that most parents do not need to share. The adopting mothers, adopting parents, open themselves to judgment at a time when it is difficult to keep their equilibrium. The adopting mother does not want to be rejected in such a fundamental way.

COMING TO A DECISION

For much of history women have not been able to choose whether to have a child or not. Yet more and more the decision to become a mother, and to enter a long-term commitment to a child, is being carefully considered by many women. The decision to adopt a child is often the final option as a way of having a child. The birth mother's decision is even more consequential, especially when many people—sometimes even the birth mother herself—think she should just place the child and get on with her life. The women (both birth and adopting mothers) in this research show what a difficult decision it was for them.

The Decision to Place

"The decision was solely mine," says Lorrie Newton. "I was looking for, you know, the perfect—everything I've ever wanted in parents—kind of thing. When we found them, actually, we [Lorrie and the baby's father] knew pretty well right off that that was the people we wanted." It seems that many of the women who plan to place their baby for adoption think they will just have the baby, place it with a family of their choice, and then do all those things they want for their life. They think that by placing their child they can do something good for someone else, help someone. However, when the actual baby is born (sometimes even before), it becomes *their* child, their particular child, to whom many give a name. Then the giving is felt more like a giving up, a loss. It seems to depend on how aware they are of the baby as their particular baby—the move from *a* baby to *my* baby. And giving up *my* baby is more difficult. Birth mothers fear this attachment, fear letting their imagination picture them in the future with the baby at their side. They fear the attachment as they begin to feel it.

Placing mothers are often alone and poor. The fathers of the babies are often not present, at least not for the long term. Sometimes the fathers are already married, or it was "just a one night stand," or they raped the woman, or they, too, are fifteen or sixteen, or they just do not want to share long-term responsibility. Hannah Eldridge, whose partner is not committed to having a child in his life, says that she did what she was supposed to do when she gave up the baby. She holds back from accepting that the child she carries within her body is her own. Hannah feels that the baby she carries is not really hers.

Hannah Eldridge. Not really mine

I nervously ring her apartment door. Hannah, small and reserved, answers with a quiet smile. She looks sad and uncomfortable. She talks quietly, hesitantly. In spite of her statement, "just never thought it would happen to me," she seems to be ambivalent about having this baby—wanting it and not wanting it. By the time I met her, Hannah had made a decision against abortion: "just too scary to think about" and she "didn't have the money." Yet she is not absolutely sure about giving the baby up for adoption. She is sure and yet not sure, until she does it. Her sister had placed her child for adoption a couple of years earlier and Hannah tells how she often talked to her sister during this pregnancy. Hannah says that her mother, too, is supportive: "She'll help me through whatever I do." Although Hannah lives with her boyfriend, there does not seem to be a long-term commitment to each other or to the coming child.

Hannah says about her pregnancy, "I wasn't as upset as I thought I would be, although it was not planned, not really wanted—a nice idea. It's weird. Just basically shock." During pregnancy, "it's like I know it's in me, but it's not really mine yet. It's just there, you know." Even after the ultrasound, "it makes it more there, just not really more mine, just more there. It is still hard for me to accept the fact that I am pregnant. Like I know I am, but I still don't think of it as mine—for giving it up, it'll be easier. It is really weird for me, like sometimes it's good and sometimes it's not. It's good to know that you have a baby and stuff even if I'm not going to keep it—it still makes me feel better for some reason." Her voice becomes more animated as she talks of feeling the baby move—"it's really neat when it happens." "Even when I see kids now," and she sees pregnant people and kids all over the place, "they're cuter, and nicer, not as bratty as I used to think they were."

In the end, Hannah places her baby with a couple who were friends of the adopting parents of her sister's baby—"to keep it in the family, so to speak." After letters and meeting together with them, Hannah says, "we gave the baby up to them. My family thought, and I thought, I was doing the right thing, for the baby and for me. It was kind of hard on my parents but they were good—really hard for them. I made a big decision and I'm more sure of myself now. I'm glad I went through it. I need to talk about it to know that it really happened. I'm not sorry I had the baby."

Everybody, that is, family, friends, and even the nurses in the hospital, agree that Hannah is doing the right thing. The birth itself was quite easy. Hannah held her baby right after he was born and a couple more times. She wrote a letter to him and hopes for some pictures in the future, but thinks it would be best to "just keep out of it." Yet, Hannah wants to talk about it, "not all the time, once in a while, just so I know I'm not denying it happened." Her boyfriend, the child's father, doesn't want to talk about it and Hannah thinks that "it is hard for him." She feels ready to start a new life—working on her relationship, going back to school, and using birth control.

"Before I had the baby," says Hannah, "it's not really my baby kind of thing, so it was easier, it was easier to do. I thought I'll just do this for someone else, so it won't be so bad when it is born. I'll just think I'm helping someone else. But when it was born . . . I mean it is yours, and I don't know . . . I'm still trying to go through whatever it is. It is not over yet. I did what I was supposed to do."

From mid-pregnancy Hannah realizes she will probably place her child for adoption, so it is easier to think that the child is not really hers. She separates herself from her baby, even if the baby is in her body. Yet, when the baby is born, she knows that this boy is *her* baby and she cannot prevent her attachment any longer. For Hannah, it seems, giving the baby up is not just a considered, rational decision: she cannot see that she has any other choice. Cathy Bishop, another placing mother, believes that, no matter what the reason, "placing a child is not easy. You're never going to forget. It's going to be always with you, always, always, and whether it was a good experience or a bad experience, like if you're forced into it or whatever, you're going to live with it for, you know, forever." Billington (1994) agrees that no woman gives away a child easily, nor does she ever forget. "The choice is not one of nonparticipation," says Maureen Connolly, "She can pretend that she was not touched or moved, but she is 'involved' even though her child is absent. She participates in the reality of the 'missed relationship,' the 'nonchance' to touch one another's lives, while at the same time realizing that her child has touched and changed her forever" (1987: 166). Women give their child up in response to what they wish for the future of the child and not for selfish reasons.

The reality of the placing mother is the disparity between the picture of what she wants for her child and what she thinks she can give her child. Most parents, in having children, create their picture as they go, so to speak—having the child, buying a house or finding an apartment, having a spare room, having a job—while developing a sense of commitment to the care of the child. The placing mother has the same ideal of the good home, but the realization of this ideal seems beyond their grasp. The placing mother feels she has nothing to give a child. She looks for the best place as home for her child. *To place* her child, is to give that child a home—a place to belong.

The Decision to Adopt

Women who become mothers by adoption usually decide to have a child years before deciding to adopt. The decision to adopt, to bring *any* child into the place of *my* child, is a big one. The woman must get to the point where having a child becomes the important part. Pregnancy and birth are given a secondary place. Women say:

Having a child was always percolating. It took us four years to realize that nothing was going to happen. Our doctor suggested adoption, but it takes time to feel ready to do that. (Karin Perry)

We started to try to have children a year after our marriage [eight years earlier] and I've had three miscarriages. Every month you have hope. Every time you ovulate, you hope that maybe *this* time... I think you get to the point where you're aching to have a child, so you accept the fact that you can't have your own. (Nel Henry)

We decided to wait until the March seminar. It gave us some time. The social worker thought we were smart to have done that—to give ourselves time. But I don't think I needed it. I mean, adoption is just the route that I wanted to go. I actually almost prefer it. So it isn't something with which we're trying to completely replace giving birth to a baby, I guess. We want children. That is what we want. (Lois Reynolds)

The decision to adopt a child as a way of becoming a mother is neither straightforward nor easy. Most women come to this decision after various setbacks in having *their own* child: medical workups, in vitro fertilization, artificial insemination, surgery, and a number of miscarriages. Although Lois says that she almost preferred to adopt, many of these women feel that their bodies let them down. Even if it is not always clear that the problem of infertility is their own, the women feel the negative edge of the definition of infertility. They are not, and perhaps never will be, pregnant. They are devastated. They are angry at themselves, at their bodies, and at life. They are "green with envy" of pregnant women or friends with babies, and do not want to be around them. Karin says, "I don't enjoy the feeling of envy I experience when I see them. You don't like to know that about yourself." They cry at the "blood in the toilet" that means another missed pregnancy. They feel incredibly sad. When Karin remarks that it is hard to think of herself as infertile, although she knows she is, her partner Gil says, "Well no, you're not. It is just that your tubes are blocked." The infertility label seems so "final. It seems to close off possibilities because it doesn't admit any gradations." The experience of infertility is a dark picture for women who want a child.

While other childless women may not have the same experience, the women I spoke to talk of their grief, their sadness, and their many disappointments. They talk of coming to terms with not being able, for whatever reason, to birth their child. "Being a mother is not being pregnant," says Jennifer Black after four months of artificial insemination. "I was trying to force something [a pregnancy] that wasn't necessary." Joan Bell, however, talks about the real pain of not being able to have her own child and of missing the pregnancy and birth experience. She feels that having a child, either a birth or adopted child, means having a stake in life, having a *whole* life. For her, having a child is not a goal; rather, "it is having life that contains the things that make for a *good* life, good for people, good for humanity, as part of my life."

Joan Bell. It gives you a stake

Joan is forty-six. Time is running out for her to exercise all the possibilities of life, which, for her, included time to have her own baby. To her, having a baby is part of a whole life, of living one's life to its fullest, of exercising the talents and capacities that one has. She does not simply "want a child in order to be a mother." For Joan, "being a mother and having a family is exercising a whole set of domestic capacities that you never exercise if you live on your own." She believes that it is totally wrong to say that a woman has missed something out of life because she doesn't have a child. Rather, "I think I'll have missed something out of *my life* if I don't. It is something that I want to do. Having a baby is not like getting some smart job. Having a baby is part of *having a life*."

Joan had eighteen attempts with artificial insemination, and when they didn't work she was terribly upset. "It's grief, more than anything else. It's the kind of anger I suspect you get when you are grieving about somebody. It's like a gap in your life, and the gap is the baby I didn't have. Simon could track when my period was coming because I would get really upset. I'd get anxious and I'd get upset. Towards the end of the time I was trying, I was really beginning to wonder, why the hell do I keep putting myself through this? I would be just so upset."

Her move to adoption is a recognition that "I'm going to do something different. It's just as valuable in its own way but it's different. And it obviously mattered to me. I would have liked to have my own child, to give birth to my own child that was kind of a part of me. So that, yes, this is something different. I think that we just had to accept that it was very unlikely that we would have our own child. Once that was accepted, then deciding to adopt was much less difficult." But Joan has a residual doubt that she will ever actually find a baby for herself, because of the shortage of babies and because of her age.

Joan was invited to attend a friend's home birth, which was "one of the nicest things that I've ever done—a most moving occasion, unmessy. I think the whole experience gave me something nothing else could have given me.

"To have a child is not an ambition, it is just a process, not something you work for, not a goal. And not something you can replace by going out and looking after children. Looking after somebody else's child is not the same thing as looking after your own child. There is a life of responsibility involved in it and a kind of decision-making that you make. How can you talk about it without sounding selfish?"

In the end Joan does not adopt a child. She says, "I have been thinking about how to live with a child. It doesn't go away. It is a huge loss. I think there's a lot of ways one might look at life, but I don't really have access to it because I don't see myself extended into the future. Not because children are extensions of yourself, but there is something about a commitment to how the future will be when your children will be in it that I think you probably don't have. It's a very emotional level, a very basic level, which you don't have when you don't have children. That's why I'm thinking about my nephew. It means thinking about a future world, a stake, a hundred years hence.

"It was definitely part of my life, but I never saw it as an ambition—not as a goal. If anything, it is a beginning of a whole process. It is like a talent: you have the capacity to exercise a skill, but you've never acquired the ground rules for exercising or the opportunity actually to exercise it. Yet you know that it is something you would be able to do. I mean I am trying to explain why there might be a sense of loss, that this is something that I could have done."

Adopting mothers, more than other mothers perhaps, sit down and talk about what mothering is for them—a stake in the future, an exercising of talents. Although many women now choose not to have a child, women who adopt want to have a child of their own in their life. Some women, like Joan, want to feel an investment in the future. Some, like Jennifer, fear that the life they want will pass them by. Others feel insecure, as if they did not fit in. For them, life without a child is lonely. Others say that not having children may make people think something is wrong with them or their marriage. They want the opportunity to love a child, to belong, to feel at peace. They want their own child. Women who adopt do so from a deep longing, a longing that only a child of their own (not necessarily through their own bodies) can satisfy. Once women open themselves up to the desire to become mother to a child and actually make the decision to adopt, they feel a gap (infertility, miscarriages, the adoption that did not happen) that nothing but a child can fill. For these women, looking after someone else's children, having nieces and nephews, even working with children, will not do. They do not want to feel like custodians. They want to feel like mothers. One can wonder how such feelings come about. Is it a sense of completeness that these women feel a child will bring, or is it a longing for something that they have always wanted in their life?

To adopt a child is to raise that child as one's own. The word *adopt* comes from the Latin *adoptāre*, meaning to choose for oneself, to desire. Yes, these women choose to adopt a child, desire a child. As a woman moves toward adoption, she wonders how to become *this* child's mother. "I think," says Joan, "that being asked what preferences you have is a most difficult question. Rather, one should be asked about what [kind of child] you can realistically think you would live with in a reasonably happy way." She goes on, "*Preferences* doesn't seem quite the right way to put it. A question like, 'What would a child get out of having us as parents?' is the way to put it. The lottery of nature, being what it is, would mean that a child might not have any of the things that we would really want for the child. The child might have loss of limbs, mental retardation, or deafness. This is life." Joan suggests that having a child is not the same as owning something for which you could order just the right size, shape, and color. Having a child, claiming a child, has to do more with having a good fit. It has to do with how a child could benefit from what the parents have to offer. While most adoptive and birth mothers report strong positive feelings for the baby right away (*love* for the baby), the adoptive mothers tend to focus on the fact that the child "is mine," rather than on the particular physical features, like "he's got my nose" (Koepke, Austin, Anglin, and Delesalle 1991). Both mothers are searching for the connection, the good fit, the belonging.

To enter the adoption experience these women need strength, as the process itself makes them feel defenseless. Jennifer puts it this way, "You feel very vulnerable. Yet I also, as I've said to my husband, I feel real strong. Like, I feel, I feel exposed—like my nerves are out there now, hanging for someone to beat around. But I also feel, 'I can do this.' " The vulnerability is inevitable. These courageous women need strength to accept and live through the wild ups and downs of the adopting process. When they reach the other side, with a child *of their own*, they deserve the respect and acknowledgment given them. They deserve the label of *wise woman* that Jennifer feels she has gained.

Adopting mothers have prepared a home for children. As Nel Henry says, they "live a lifestyle of a couple waiting to have a child," or like Karin Perry, "here we are with a three-bedroom house, well settled, and the things we like to do I think would be great for kids to do." Outwardly these adopting mothers seem to have it made: they are women with good incomes and supportive partners. I met the women in this research—teachers, doctors, social workers, professors, bank managers, nurses, small business owners, technicians—in their three-bedroom, middle-class homes, in good, quiet neighborhoods, with a park across the street, and with backyards ready for playing children. These homes, symbols of solid families, stand ready, waiting—ready as the ironing board set up in the empty room across the hall from the master bedroom. These women, capable and eager images of the Good Mother, stand ready too. Because they do not want to be at home alone they endure the incredible pain that comes from desperately wanting a child, as well as the vulnerability of waiting to be chosen. On the one hand, the adopting mother has the home that she wants, but on the other hand, she feels like she stands outside that home, "always on the outside kind of looking in." She stands ready to claim a child and hopes that, before long, a birth mother will choose her.

PRESENCE AND ABSENCE

Birth mothers experience the presence of the child in their bodies, and that presence stays with them in the child's absence. Living with the absent child is a chronic state, given to remembering, caring, and loving. It is also acute, with "great sharpness and severity at those times when the presence of other things make [the] absence so keenly, intensely felt" (Connolly 1987: 167). Adopting mothers experience the absence of the child in their bodies as well—the hope that "every time you ovulate, maybe *this* time." They see babies everywhere and feel their arms empty. Where does this sense of emptiness come from—is it biological or social? Or is it both of these and even more—a spiritual desire and a cultural expectation?

The Presence of the Absent Child

Cathy Bishop did not have access to open adoption when she relinquished her child at sixteen, and she wonders about the openness of open adoption. She does not know where her child is and wonders how she could handle it if she did. She says, "She's been in the back of my mind for so long, she's there but she's really not. She pops up, and I kind of wonder how she is doing and what she looks like. I wonder, if I was to see her would I recognize her?" But still in the distance of anonymity she is involved with her child: "she's been in the back of my mind for so long."

Whether it is the child's birthday that reminds the birth mother, or seeing other children who might be the age of the placed child, or a sister who is pregnant, or a friend who adopts a baby, there is a recognition of the absent child. The child is remembered. Lois Reynolds, an adopting mother, tells of her sister who gave up a child for adoption thirteen years previously. There is never an October that goes by when Lois's sister does not think of him. Lois says that when her sister "heard we were getting a baby through adoption, she applied to have her name in the adoption registry in case her child wanted to find her. I think it was really good for her to see us get a child. Like her wonderful favor was repaid now—has come around full circle." Allison Decker (another placing mother whose child was placed through closed adoption) has celebrated her daughter Cindy's birthday for ten years now. She has a bundle of cards that she hopes to give Cindy at some distant date. Allison's own mother always sends a yellow rose to Allison on the birthday of her absent child. With open adoption, the birth mother may send presents and cards, may talk on the phone with the adopting parents, may even attend the birthday party. Often, however, she celebrates alone. Yet no matter how the day of birth is celebrated, the day is remembered—by the birth mother and perhaps even by the birth grandmother. We begin to see the extent of the absent child's presence.

Sally Corbett. It'll never go away . . . never

"I was feeling kind of yucky and I went to the doctor and he told me that I was six months pregnant and I had no idea. Cause I still had girl's thing happen. I didn't believe him even when he did an ultrasound. I didn't gain any weight until I think I was about eight and a half months. I had no idea. The first time I knew was when he kicked me. And I'm like 'holy . . . what's going on down there.' And you'd see my shirt like popping. It was neat though. I finally believed the doctor when the baby kicked me. When the baby came popping out everyone was surprised that he was so big [eight pounds, four ounces].

"I told my mom about my pregnancy and we kept it a secret for a while, didn't say anything. Then she told my grandparents and my aunts and uncles. Only two of my friends know, and that's it." Sally has never known her own father, and she says her baby's father does not care. "He had other kids behind my back."

She tells of how she chose the adopting parents. "I was looking through the files and none of them appealed to me. And then I opened up *their* file and they looked so happy. The pictures, that's what caught my eye first. They had big smiles on their faces and in every picture I looked at they were so happy and seemed so loving. I read their letter to the birth mother, recognizing the hard choice I was making and saying that whatever they can do they'd do to help me. And then I met them and I knew right then. They just seemed so nice and so caring. And the first time I saw them they cried—they were so happy that someone had picked them.

"It didn't bother me until the day before the social worker came for me to sign the papers giving me ten days to change my mind. Then it got harder. When they took him home it was the hardest. I cried and cried and cried.

"A couple months ago, I was driving down the street by myself, and it just hit that he was gone and that was it. I just started to cry. I think about him a lot and I want to take him home with me but I know I can't. The adoption was final on Friday. We went to court on Friday—that was pretty tough. I thought it would be a lot easier, but it was so cold, like the judge just seemed so cold. He just kind of signed his name on the paper and stamped it. And that was it. And after that I was pretty upset, but I'll live with it.

"The good things were that I brought this beautiful boy into the world and that he'll always have a happy home, but then the bad thing is that I took the loss. Sometimes I think I did the right thing and other times I think no, I think he'd be better with me because in my head I always think no one could treat him the way that I could. I'm his real mum.

"I know if I ever got pregnant again, I wouldn't even have a second thought of giving the baby up. It would stay with me and I wouldn't even think of having an abortion. I said that to my mum, 'If I ever got pregnant again and it was by accident, I would never even have any other doubt in my head for to keep the baby.' I think once he was born and I saw what kind of a miracle he was, and he's just . . . the best thing ever. . . . I want to do whatever I can to have all the money and have a nice house and a really good family, like a really good husband, so that when I have kids my baby will have just as good of a home as what the other baby has. I want to be able to give him or her whatever I possibly could."

It is the embodied presence of the child that makes this experience so difficult and causes mothers to wonder where the best place is for their baby. This wonder is shown in Sally's conflicted thinking that her baby would be better with her because she is his "real mum." But then she says, "They are probably treating him ten times better than anybody could ever. But I always think, well I could give him this, and I could do this, but I know that he'll have such a happy home and they love him so much. It's just unreal." We hear how birth mothers struggle with desire for their child to have what they think they need for a good life, and the desire in themselves to give the child what they have to give. Many of the birth mothers love being pregnant, they love the feelings of their child inside. As Lorrie Newton says, "it's just amazing. I can lay there for hours, put my hand on it, wait for it to kick." Some feel that they know their child—when hungry, when sleeping or awake, if it liked music, or didn't like smoke. "I feel like I've got a kid. He'll be awake from two to four in the morning. So I'm up with him, you know, talking at my stomach. 'What do you want? Are you hungry?' It's total, a total attachment."

The experience of presence of the baby is what makes it so difficult. "I break down and cry and think, 'it's my baby, how can I do this?' " Some mothers feel that it is through their pregnancy, and their experience of the baby inside, that they learn about themselves, they realize what life is, and what is important in life. Lorrie describes how she changed through the connection to the growing child within.

Lorrie Newton. I've really felt life

"I used to think there was unlimited time for everything. You know. I didn't have to get a job now because, you know, I can always do that later. I didn't really care about today. But now I do. Now every day is kind of special—even a tree, it used to be just a tree but now it's a living thing. I take a lot more appreciation for life. I guess it's the first time I've really felt life. It's inside, and I can feel it moving and stuff, and it just made me a lot more aware of everything around me.

"I didn't like kids very much. I used to sort of look at them and, you know, stick my nose up. Never going to have a kid. But now I look at them and say, 'Wow. They're so cute.' I love kids. I just think they're really funny. Kids are funny and kids don't care about anything. I can just watch them for hours. Run around and scream at the top of their lungs for no reason. It's great. Totally uninhibited.

"The decision to give up my baby sort of made me realize that there's a lot of people in my life that I really care about, that I don't tell them I care. I sort of kept these feelings bottled up for years. Now I'm realizing there's not enough time. You should tell people how you feel. So I called my granny and told her I loved her. I don't remember ever telling her that before. So I had to call her. She thinks I'm getting kind of weird. I'm becoming a lot more, not emotional, but I'm letting my feelings show a lot more. I don't know, I think it's just realizing how precious life is now. And thinking about the people that could . . it's a horrible thing to say but my granny could die tomorrow. I'll never have told her I loved her and I thought about that and I thought, 'That's horrible.' So I started telling my friends that I do care about them. I try not to be so cold, because normally I'm kind of reserved and I don't tell people that I care about them. I just assume they know that.

"I am going to try to build up my life after this. It's going to be kind of tough, I'm sure, for a while. I don't know if I'll even be able to work for a while, because it's probably going to take a little bit out of my head. Might kind of lose it after giving up the baby, but I feel a lot better knowing where the baby is. I think I'm going to Toronto. I just want to go somewhere where nothing's going to remind me of the pregnancy, or the baby, or anything. So that I can get over it, easier, faster. And try and start working and get my mind on other things. And no one's going to talk to me about it all the time. People here, when they heard I was giving up the baby, they treat me like I am a china doll, you know, 'Oh be careful what you say.' "

Other women, who do not describe this kind of strong relationship with their growing fetus, still look back on the pregnancy as a time of change in their life—a time of growing up or settling down or paying attention to life differently than they had previously. They learn about who they are, and who they are not. Lorrie talks of building her own life, being closer to friends and family, being more open with affection and love. Sally says she is more willing to go to her friends when they need her. Hannah talks of being more confident, more determined to get her education and move forward with her life.

The presence of the child for the birth mother is an embodied experience. So, too, for the adopting mother. Although Sandelowski calls the adopting women's experience "the disembodied nature of childwaiting" (1993: 181), the bodily experience is very powerful. The devastation and grief of the "blood in the toilet" is a concrete, bodily reminder that the child is not there. Her arms are empty. The glimmer of hope that adopting mothers feel when they are chosen by a birth mother is like "one's period is a day late." But being chosen is only a glimmer, and as such contains the fear of yet another horrific disappointment, so that some, like Charlotte, can only say "I feel like I'm going to throw up."

Hands Tied Down

The presence of the child in the life of the adopting woman is made real by the match, which is the choice made by the birth mother. Like the ultrasound examination for the pregnant woman, the first glimpse of the real child for the adopting woman is when the birth mother chooses her. A good match may indicate some similarity between the birth mother and the adopting mother—interests, likes and dislikes. Some adopting mothers think the birth mother "could be a good neighbor" or "is like a sister." Some, like Charlotte, might say, "I'm crazy about her." At the same time, the good match has another dimension: the remarkable difference between the women, in terms of home, job, money, security, partners, family, and so on. Whose fantasy is played out in the desire for a good match? In this match, the players are at opposite ends of the social playing field. It is a game in which only one team can really score and the birth mother seems to hold the trump to determine the winner.

During the birth mother's pregnancy, the adopting mother gets as close as she dares. The adopting mother, like the placing mother, holds herself back for she knows the risks of letting the child come too close. She knows that she might yet lose the child. She may want to touch the birth mother's belly, but that is as close as she gets. The risks are there. She holds the baby at arm's length. The child is a fragile presence for the adopting mother. At the same time as she needs to protect herself from being too close to the child, she wants to open herself to the child. "I'm scared," says Nel Henry, "I'm concerned about how I am going to bond with this baby. And about the open adoption part. Because I don't have a relationship with this child yet to keep me kind of secure." She wants to keep in touch with the birth mother to keep her secure. Yet, she must "prepare for the worst," says Connie Hancock. Even when she is chosen the adopting mother is cautious.

It is a very long pregnancy when a woman reaches for the baby with her hands tied down! The adopting woman's "pregnancy" is not just nine months—it could be nine years. "Four years ago," says Nel, "would have been a good time for a child." And then, even when the child does come, one wonders "will I always be his mother?" The adoptive mother knows that this child, while hers and finally in her arms, is never just hers. The reality of one child with two mothers sinks in (Billington 1994).

Nel Henry. Will I always be his mother?

"Every month you hope, every time you ovulate you hope that maybe this is the time. I have twinges of jealousy when I see a pregnant woman walking down the street. I can't go any further, personally, until I have a baby. An adopted baby. Because then I think I'd be a lot more at peace with myself, like, I sort of fit in. Then maybe I won't be so upset about not getting pregnant."

Before the birth, Nel thinks that the friendship with the birth mother will be very short-lived. It is a friendship with a purpose. She says, "I don't want to get really emotionally involved as a friendship—just respect, and trust, and understanding of each other. I'm very comfortable meeting her. I really want to meet her. I just don't want her to be a part of my life afterwards, cause I think that it would really be hard for her to deal with. She needs to grieve and she needs to end that part of her life to get on with the rest of her life. I like open adoption because I can tell this child everything that she or he needs to know. I've met the woman, there is not a mystery like 'who is this person?'

"We got a phone call saying we had been picked by a birth mom, and we met her and her grandmother. I was very nervous. Very, very nervous. And it was hard to find a place where you could speak and get to know each other, that was neutral. We chose a restaurant, which was probably a good choice for that time. Unfortunately there was this person sitting beside us who kept looking over. She's probably wondering, 'what the heck are these people talking about?' I'm sure it made no sense to anybody who didn't really know what we were doing. Because it was almost like we were being interviewed but we were also doing some interviewing. It went really well. She had her questions written down. We had our questions written down. And we asked each other the questions. I think we arranged to meet again after that meeting was over. She phoned and we phoned. Because she was concerned that we wouldn't like her, which just blows my mind away. I am the one, we are the ones that are on . . . sort of being checked out, I think. But she felt the same, that she was being checked out. It was a go.

"I just felt that this baby was going to be born any minute, and it was all that I could think about. I was just totally engulfed in this delivery and this child. I would talk to the birth mother. I would call her, you know, she would call me—we had an ongoing relationship. We went shopping together. I was still fairly cautious about what to buy because I wasn't one hundred percent convinced the baby would come home with us. But I wanted to see her, to touch her belly. When I talked to her, I felt reassured. It kept us in her mind, so she wouldn't forget us.

"The baby was born on a Sunday. I found out Monday at work and I phoned Greg right away. We went to the hospital with flowers. She was actually still on the high stage at that point, and we were able to go into the intensive care, her and I, only. She said, 'Well, you hold him first' and I held him. We went to the hospital every day, and saw her and saw him, and it was getting progressively harder for her. And I was getting really panicky because I thought she was going to change her mind, because the longer she was in the hospital, the longer he was in the hospital. The more time they were spending together, the closer they were getting. It was hard. Friday was the day that he was going to be discharged. She signed the papers in the morning. She had asked that we be there at noon, and at four o'clock she still hadn't gone.

"That was probably the hardest thing I think I've ever had to do. Greg was crying, I was crying, she was crying. Everyone was just very very upset. It was such a happy moment but . . . As soon as Greg brought up the car seat, just everybody lost it. So she dressed him and we put him in the car seat. She came downstairs with us. I was still crying when I got in the car. I was in the back seat with him and just in *awe*. You're in shock, you know, because you're all of a sudden . . . I think when you're pregnant you have the nine months, which does make a difference because you feel that there's more reality.

"I think she was very surprised at her own feelings because she said, 'I just thought I'd have this baby and give it to you and that will be it.' You know, she had no idea. She's a very mature nineteen, I think, because in some ways she had thought of a lot of things. I think she had made a very wise decision and she had all the reasons why she'd made the decision.

"The minute I saw him I knew he was ours, which was very very strange. Because there were all kinds of babies in that room, and the second I saw him, I knew it was him. I mean, I knew who we were looking for, there was just this invisible string, you know. He wasn't a stranger. Maybe because I liked his look.

"Most people are quite afraid of birth mothers, I think. I know my mom and Greg's family are quite concerned that something's going to happen and she's going to take the baby away and something like that. I have to trust, I think, to let, sort of, just kind of let that go, and maybe we're just fortunate, because I don't feel threatened by her. But I certainly feel her love for him. I know how much I feel for Timothy and I know what she's missing. And I can imagine, I can only imagine how much loss, especially at Christmastime, how much loss she's feeling right now. I know how many smiles and joys he's brought into our life, and she's missing that. And I know she made her decision, but what a hard decision! And I really feel for her. I think I mentioned before some fear about the future. And that's more down the road, like, you know, five, ten years down the road, you know, when he's old enough to know. Sandy and her family are going to be part of our lives—at different levels throughout our life. Because I've met her grandmother and I've met her grandfather, I've met her mother, I've met her aunts and her uncles and her cousins. I've met them all. They've met us. It is hard. Because I really wanted to keep it fairly low-key and it was O.K. with her mother and her grandmother, but when I started meeting aunts and uncles and cousins I said, 'I'm getting out of here!' You still want to keep your distance, you know. On one hand, I want to just hug her and let her come for Christmas and, on the other hand, I just think, 'No! Stop!'

"Do I want to do this again? I hear women say that they have a painful delivery and you forget about the pain. But I haven't forgotten about my pain yet—it's just surprising. I thought I would have but . . .

As the adopting mother reaches out to claim the child—not a stranger but the "one we were looking for"—her hands and heart become untied. Yet the fear of getting too close is still there. Although the women are ready, they anticipate the fear of being disappointed. Yet they are not always prepared for the intensity of the pain.

MOTHERING PAIN

It seems rather strange to speak of pain in speaking of adopting mothers, for we often think only of the pain of childbirth itself. Even with the placing mothers, it is not the pain of the birth itself that is most profound. For these women the pain comes before and after the birth of the child. For placing mothers the pain of the separation from the child—symbolized by the signing of the papers—is in some ways bigger and certainly more long-lasting than birthing pain.

Signing the Papers

Lorrie Newton placed her child for adoption. She talks of being treated like a china doll, a fragile, easily shattered person. She does not like it. But the china doll image does give a sense of the ongoing fragility of these women, a fragility that may last for years. For many mothers who decide to place their babies for adoption, the extent of their pain is unforeseen. They prepare for the placement with their minds. They do not realize that their hearts are not so easily disciplined. They do not know, ahead of time, the depth of their connection to the child and to their mothering feelings. Sally Corbett's words show the extent of the pain: "Before the baby was born, I didn't think it would be as hard as it was. I thought it would be a piece of cake—that he'd be born and that would be it. But it wasn't at all.

Before I held him, he was just a ball in my belly, and it didn't really mean as much. But the first time I held him, like, 'No way, I'm not going to do it.' But I didn't really say anything except to my mum. I said, 'I don't know if I want to do this.' " Later she found out that everyone knew by the look on her face. "The adoptive parents came and saw me that day, and they said that they knew. And I said, 'Well, how can you tell?' and they said, 'We can just tell by looking at you.' But I told them that 'even though I do have second thoughts, he'll still be going home with you.' "

The women wept as they told me of their experience. The pain they remember is not so much the pain of labor and birth itself (although it too was intense), but the nagging, lingering pain of the long-term separation from their child, which formally signing the papers put in motion. In addition to the separation pain of labor and birth—becoming two separate beings—birth mothers are faced with a gulf of separation that may be forever present. Mothering pain is present for all the mothers—those who birth, those who adopt, and those who place the child, who perhaps suffer the most. In placing her child in the kind of home she wants this child to have, the birth mother has the pain of giving away the day-to-day mothering way of life.

"I remember leaving him: I am lingering at the window of his nursery watching him move in his sleep. My fingers are on the glass and I whisper 'goodbye, baby' and I'm crying very quietly and feeling an ache—not only in my throat but in my heart, in my bones, that will be there, more or less intensely, for as long as I live" (Connolly 1987: 164). We know that it is proper for babies to have the lives they deserve, but it is equally proper, says Maureen Connolly, to respect the birth mother's unending wondering about her child: "She gave, but is unable to forget; her son belongs to other parents now: He is theirs in a way that he can never be hers. Yet he is hers in a way that he can never be theirs. This is the fundamental and apparently unresolvable contradiction of the meaning of adoption" (Connolly 1987: 164). With open adoption the grief and pain of the giving mother is acknowledged. The conspiracy of silence, which suggests that the birth mother just forgets it and starts over, is broken (Howe 1990). Birth mothers do grieve the loss of the child, and it may be a continuing loss because the child is still living. It is the grief of the unbroken cord, a loss that may increase over time (Winkler and van Keppel 1984; Blanton and Deschner 1990). This grief, well named as shadow grief (Lauderdale and Boyle 1994), is carried by these mothers as though nothing had happened, that child was never born and that they were not mothers. Speaking about their grief may be the first step for birth mothers in living through it.

Jesse Abbott placed her baby boy for adoption when he was seven months old. Jesse, struggling with the possibility of adoption since Teddy's birth, was the best mother she could be those first months, yet in the end decided that adoption was best for her baby and for herself. Her mothering pain is palpable.

Jesse Abbott. My heart broke wide open

"I was sixteen years old and I'd been in a relationship with my boyfriend for about two years. We used a condom, and it didn't even break. My aunt had instilled in me 'protection, protection, you've got to protect yourself,' so I was shocked when I found out I was pregnant. I lived with my single mom and my older brother. I was concerned about telling my mom because she's had a couple of abortions and I was against them and I thought she was going to make me have one. In September I went to school [for pregnant teenagers] with adoption in my mind. Yet, I looked at all the other girls there. They had a lot less than I did, and a lot less support. I thought, well, if they can keep, so can I. My boyfriend knew my plans of keeping and he thought that will be great.

"The labor itself was pain like you've never experienced before—an atrocious pain coming every two minutes, every minute, every thirty seconds, and I wasn't breathing properly. I was hyperventilating. My boyfriend didn't come in the labor room with me, but my mom stayed with me. I came home with the baby on a Sunday, and so that Monday my brother was in school, my mom went to work, so I was left home alone with this baby. I didn't know what to do. Like I babysat before, but I had to feed him, bathe him, burp him. 'How do you bathe him properly?' 'What happens if he starts coughing and he chokes, what do I do?' I was scared because I was alone.

"I first went down to the adoption agency when he was about five weeks old. I looked at some files. I chose a family, but I wasn't sure if I wanted to carry on with the adoption. The pain that I was going through trying to make that decision, like 'I love him dearly, I don't want to have to do this, but realistically I can't give him the life that I wanted him to have.' I was trying so hard to try to make things work. I was going to school full-time and in the summer I managed to get a part-time job. Come September I was back in school. I tried a regular high school and with him that didn't go over at all.

"Then he was in the hospital for about five or six days. We were at a bus terminal and I was holding him just kind of under the bum, not a good grip like you're supposed to have on his back. He was about six months old, and I was just getting off the bus to transfer on to another bus and I was fixing his diaper bag on my shoulder and I had turned my head for a second and this kid was trying to catch the bus and ran right into us and at the same time Teddy stretched. I didn't have a good grip on him, so Teddy fell out of my arms and he fell down and hit his head on the concrete. One of the passengers had seen it and came out to help me. Teddy seemed okay. But they wanted to do X-rays just in case. I called my mom and as soon as I heard her voice on the line I just burst into tears. I was under the age of eighteen but I was living on my own after going to the Appeal Board to get my own place. I had full custody of my son, and the nurse came and told my mom that she had to sign the papers for the hospital. I had social workers in my room the first few days I was there—enquiring into what had happened. I thought, 'I'm sitting there, I've spent every hour that I had in the rocking chair, and if he had a bad night, I slept with him on me.' I had these people coming in asking me if I beat my child. They treated me like dirt there. And then I ended up having a home study come in, just to follow up and see how he's doing after his stay in the hospital.

"About a month later after all this I thought, you know, 'This is too much. I can't do this any more. I can't live on my own, and try and raise him, I'm living in a dream world, trying to make it something that it is not.' Like I admitted that I was a young, frustrated mother. I was going to school full-time, had a part-time job working weekends, and my mom was babysitting on the weekends. I saw him for maybe two hours a day during the week and at weekends. I wasn't raising him. Everybody else but me was raising him. His father wasn't in the picture to help raise him. That's not the life I wanted for him. I wasn't enjoying parenting any more. I couldn't do it like I thought I could and he was suffering because of it. I was thinking that this is not right, this is not the way a child should be raised, I can't do this to him, I'm not happy, he's not happy, he's suffering because of it.

"I decided to place Teddy for adoption when he was over seven months old. When the adopting parents came to pick him up I carried him down the stairs. His dad had come to be with us. I am just torn up inside and Teddy's just laughing away. I remember standing at the door. I was holding him. Pat [the adopting mother] kind of got her arms half-open, not totally outstretched. She's kind of got them half waiting and ready and I've got my hold a little tighter. I don't want to let go. I gave him a big kiss and everything, 'Mommy loves you.' As soon as I hand him over I start crying and then Pat starts crying. She gives me a hug when she was holding him and I say, 'Just let him know that I love him and I'll always love him' and she said, 'oh yeah.' She's just bawling away, and she says, 'He'll always know that, there's nothing that we won't tell him and you'll see him in time. We'll send you pictures regularly.'

"You know, my whole life was walking out the door.

"So they walked out to the car. I went into the apartment and there's a window. I was watching. I hadn't stopped crying and I looked out the window and saw them pulling away. It was dark outside. It was nighttime. I remember the last thing that I saw was her leaning over the passenger seat fixing the blanket on him, making sure he was all comfortable, fixing the blanket. Then he went around the corner. I just stared there for a while. There was nothing outside and there was nothing in the apartment. I was just numb."

Jesse talked of this experience for hours, remembering small intimate details. She asked to talk to me: she wanted to share her experience. The decision to place is encouraged by a social and cultural image of the good family, mother, father, income, home, stability—providing everything for a child. With this image there is the suspicion that the young birth mother is not capable—a suspicion acted out by hospital personnel in Jesse's case. She began to agree that she was not the capable mother she wanted to be. When a child is placed, it is important for the birth mother to acknowledge it, to share the experience with others, especially with future partners. Her experience of placing needs to be integrated into her ongoing life (Ryan 1990). These young women need the opportunity to share their experience and have it valued and appreciated. Who will listen to their stories? Who will ask?

Ripped out of Your Arms

The mothering pain that adopting mothers experience is also incredible. It is different than birthing pain, more diffuse, more long-lasting. It is not confined to the twelve or twenty-four hours of labor, but comes before the child's birth and lasts for a long time after the birth. While adopting mothers may experience the severe pain of miscarriage, painful medical examinations, or procedures like in vitro fertilization, they also experience the fear-based pain of having the birth mother change her mind. The birth mother may change her mind before birth or after, after one day or nine, or even after months. She might even turn up years later to claim her child. Through childbirth pain and its tumultuous rhythm, the mother and child are separated from an incredible physical bond—the baby is thrust into life as a separate being and they end up separate but close. In adoption pain there is no identifiable rhythm, no distinguishable beginning or end. The child of an adopting mother is already a separate being, separate from her. The pain of adoption is the pain of connecting to the baby and the birth mother, and the fear of separation from them. This is what adopting mothers say about their pain:

She can have three babies and I can't have one. I think all these things we are going through now will all disappear as soon as we have a baby. Just like we say about delivery. You know, how horrible it is. But as soon as you've had the baby you forget what you went through. I think that's probably how I'll feel. (Lois Reynolds)

I had everything. I had the laparoscopy, the biopsies, I had everything, and I said to my husband, "You know, this is really stupid. I mean, as much as I want to have a child, I don't have to have one this way. This is stupid." (Jennifer Black)

We had to come to this willingness to accept the risk that this child could be taken away from us—there might be a match and the birth mother might change her mind and decide to keep the baby, or she may decide she didn't want us to have the baby either before she gave birth or before the ten days were up, which would be awful. You have to accept the risk. I mean, really, your heart will be broken. (Karin Perry)

The vulnerability I think you have is that you're sort of . . . nothing is signed and sealed and written in stone. I mean, like you're virtually at everybody's mercy. That has to be, that's the only way you can do it. The mother has ten days after the baby is born. Even if she's chosen you and the baby's born, it still doesn't mean anything, really, it doesn't. You know it's a joyous, happy time but you're still on edge. You feel very vulnerable. (Connie Hancock)

It's really frightening. You go through the days of sheer hell. You know you are bonding with this child. This child is yours. You've decided it is yours, and then she [the birth mother] rips it out of your arms. That is how I would feel it would be like. And that would break my heart. You have to be pretty strong about the whole thing and hope you don't lose your mind in the whole process. (Jennifer Black)

For some women the pain of being chosen and being rejected is like a death. Barbara, who planned to adopt using a private lawyer to facilitate the adoption, tells her experience.

Barbara Campbell. He was ours

It is a luxurious home, with a fountain in the front hall and a musical doorbell that announces my arrival. Barbara, a soft-spoken teacher, wants another child. Sam is seven. For about four years this family waited for another child. Barbara had two miscarriages.

They met Jocelyn on Wednesday, the day after the baby boy was born. Although teary at the time, Jocelyn said she was very confident that she was doing the right thing in putting her baby up for adoption. She had just turned eighteen. Although it was a hard thing for her to do, in her heart she felt it was the right thing. She couldn't provide for him. When the hospital staff realized Jocelyn had decided to place her child for adoption, they congratulated her and said it was a wonderful decision—so unselfish of her to do that. It was good that she could complete the goals that she had set for herself, finish her high school and then go to university to get her education. She had all these plans that she realized she could not carry out and really give the baby what was best for him. It was because both Barbara and Mark were teachers that she chose them over two other couples. Jocelyn was thought to be very confident that she was making the right decision. Jocelyn left the hospital on Thursday. Earlier she had wanted Barbara to come back that morning, Thursday, to visit with her, but then had the social worker phone Barbara to say "Please don't come. It would be too hard." On Friday, Barbara and Mark went to the hospital and took baby Daniel home. "He's here and he's ours. It was just an instant, like with my own. Identical!"

Barbara felt there really wasn't going to be any problem. They honestly thought that if she was going to change her mind it would have been before she left the hospital. They were not prepared. "The minute you bring the baby home, you just think, okay, now it is all a technicality. We just have to wait for the papers to be signed and wait the ten days. You know, you're on pins and needles but you don't really feel that it's going to backfire."

Monday morning the lawyer called Barbara. Jocelyn had changed her mind. "Jocelyn came to the house to pick him up. The lawyers felt maybe if she came and saw that he was being well looked after and cared for she might rethink her decision. She brought a friend with her, the one that was in the delivery room. They just stood in the kitchen. I was upstairs. When I came down, Mark asked me if I had brought Daniel down, and I said, 'No.' He went up and got him. She gave me a hug, you know, and kept saying that she was so sorry, that she just couldn't live with her decision, and she said maybe had she not seen him, it would have been different. But her doctor said it wouldn't have mattered.

"Our mistake was telling Sam that, you know, this baby was the one that we were going to adopt. So on that Monday we took him out of school so he could say goodbye. There was no way he could come home from school and find out that this baby's gone. But he did not want to say goodbye. It was hard for him to even look at him, and now he will not say his name, he refers to 'you-know-who.' He won't use his name any more. After the baby was taken away we got the dog. We got it for Sam. First, like he knew I was pregnant and knew the baby died. Then we got a baby and he was thrilled and that was taken away. We thought, well, at least if we get him a dog, it is his. We did not even tell him we were picking up this puppy. He closed his eyes, and I brought this puppy and put it in his lap and he was shocked. He said to me after, 'Well, at first, Mom, I kind of thought maybe it was Daniel, that maybe Daniel had come back to live with us.'

"I still have his baby pictures. We had those taken at the hospital, and I've been meaning to send them to her, the birth mom. I just haven't been able to do it yet. I want to send them to her and let her know not that we're angry or anything, but . . . I think it is fair to let her know that it hurt. It wasn't just her and us involved. She involved a lot of people in this kind of decision. When I do send the pictures to her and write her a letter, I might ask her if once in a while she would send us a picture.

"It is not like a miscarriage," says Barbara, "it is like a death."

Barbara's experience is the one adopting mothers fear—that once the decision has been made the birth mother will change her mind. Mothers have a way of attaching to a baby very quickly when the heart is ready, even if one guards against it. And like Barbara, when the child is no longer in one's arms, one is left sad, angry, and in pain. Here Barbara is the one to experience the absence—she is the one who asks for pictures.

Some people seem to feel that it is better for some women to place their babies than keep them. Some healthcare professionals are unsure of how much they should be involved in the decision, from fear that persuasion would lead in a certain direction, to a decision that the birth mother would not be able to live with (Mander 1991a, b). Before the birth, a birth mother's decision cannot be firm, as there is the potential that the birth experience and seeing the baby may affect her decision. Before the birth, the mother can feel sure that she has made a good, rational decision. Yet, when the child arrives, she may decide as Pauline did, to take the baby home herself. Approximately a quarter of the birth mothers who plan to place will end up changing their minds.

Pauline Earl. Changing my mind [1]

Pauline planned all along to give her baby up for adoption. From an earlier marriage she had given birth to two other children. There was Melinda, who had just turned two. Chuck, who was born four months prematurely, died one hour after his birth. Neither Pauline nor her partner Manfred felt ready for another baby. "I'm just not ready. I'm only nineteen. I don't need any more babies. He's twenty-seven and he's had a life. I just need a life. I never had much of a life, sixteen getting pregnant with her, seventeen having her, seventeen having my second one. And Manfred's not ready neither because he just . . . when he got together with me he became a instant dad with Melinda. Moneywise I'm not ready. If I was older, and Melinda was older, I'd probably keep this baby. But I'm only . . . I just turned nineteen last month.

"It's an open adoption, so it's not too bad. They gave us about six files to choose from. And Manfred helped me. I picked them, but I wanted his decision on it too. We met the family at a shopping mall about two months before the birth. I was really nervous at first. I promised myself not to smoke in front of them, but I was so nervous. They're nice people, they like kids. They were going to adopt another one, but the mother changed her mind. So they had their hopes up and said they don't want their hopes built up now again. I kept telling them that I'm giving the baby away, I'm giving the baby. They said the other girl said the same thing. But I can't change my mind."

At the meeting, Pauline and Manfred worked out some of the details of the adoption with the adopting family. "I get three days with the baby. Whoever out of my family or Manfred's family wants to come and see it, they can come. But I don't think I can be there on the third day when they come and pick the baby up. I don't, oh I don't think I can do that part. I asked for pictures every six months. They agreed on visitation rights, and only in the teen years if he wants to see or meet me he can. But I don't think I can do it any earlier than that."

Pauline's family understood her decision—and it was not an easy one. "I'm just scared I'll change my mind, 'cause I don't want to change my mind, but it has crossed my mind a couple of times. It'll be kind of hard to see your baby there, just pictures. But it's better than nothing, I guess. We're going to write a letter to the baby and she'll understand the reason why I gave her up and that I love her and everything—it's not that I didn't love her."

This pregnancy was difficult. Pauline had to have a suture put into her cervix to keep it closed. When she went into labor, the doctor had difficulty removing the stitch and gave Pauline a general anesthetic to get the stitch out. "I was going to have natural childbirth. But as soon as they cut the stitch, I started bleeding. When I woke up I asked when I was going to have my baby, 'cause I didn't know I was having a C-section. They said, 'You already had your baby.' " Before Pauline saw the baby she told the nurse that she planned to place him for adoption. Then she started to change her mind. "A boy. He's going to be my last. But what I thought of right away was my second baby. We thought it was a girl through the whole pregnancy. I told everyone I was giving him up for adoption and then I changed my mind, but I wouldn't say nothing until Manfred said it first." Pauline tried to contact the adopting family to tell them that she had changed her mind, but ended up telling the counselor at the adoption agency. "I just feel sorry for them [the adopting family] 'cause they were turned down with another one. That's what bothers me."

Ryan looks like Manfred and shares his blood type—Manfred is the father. As soon as Pauline and Ryan were out of the hospital, they started visiting around and taking him to the bingo to show him off. Keeping Ryan has been a challenge. Although Manfred's family assures them that "you can always afford a baby," raising two children is a financial burden when neither parent is working. They have no doubts about their decision to keep Ryan. "He makes us too happy now. I think we just thought of losing him. Like a stillborn, it would be the same thing."

The pregnancy and the birth of the child change the birth mother's experience of her previous decision. The embodied presence of the child before birth and the reality of the child after birth have an impact. Other circumstances—such as the sex, the blood type proving fatherhood, as well as the support from one's family—can change the balance so that the original decision is overturned. In open adoption, where the relationship between the birth mother and the adopting mother begins during the pregnancy, the birth mother worries about the adopting mother when she contemplates changing her mind. "There's a lot of people out there that can't have babies and here I'm getting pregnant every year. That's what I think of—what they're going through," says Pauline. Sally says that her commitment to the adopting parents is what holds her to the decision to place: "It was just because I knew the parents so well and they were so nice that I couldn't hurt them that way. And he'd have such a better life with them. And I could go on with my life and eventually I'd have kids, again, someday—then I'd be ready." The reality and nature of adoption, especially open adoption, is that giving and receiving means change, adaptation, and unsureness of the decision, which is extremely difficult for all parties. The mothering pain for one woman is associated with not being able to birth and for the other it is not being able to mother—for both it is like a death.

BELONGING WITH

"Becoming a mother necessarily alters a woman's pre-existing self-concept, says Kathryn Rabuzzi (1994: ix). Nel Henry, an adopting mother, agrees that one's ordinary experience is gone: "It's affected everything. You can't do anything anymore, spontaneously or quickly—don't go out." How does a woman take on motherhood? We say that adoption is for the child. But in saying this there is the danger of denying the reality of experience of the mothers. If we deny the experience of mothers, we make adoption a fiction—as if childbirth did not occur at all. If we consider adoption to be only for the child, we may deny that the birth mother was ever pregnant or that the adopting mother did not give birth to the child herself (Rabuzzi 1994). In open adoption this fiction cannot occur. The adopting mother is often at the birth. She sees where her baby comes from. She sees the birth mother push the baby into the world. She sees the birth mother reach for her baby. Even if she does not attend the birth, she knows the birth mother and her family. Charlotte Elias, an adopting mother, says, "It is hard to say *my* baby, it's usually *the* baby. Because I can feel her pain. I can feel her love. I also feel directly responsible for her sadness." When Nel Henry left the hospital with Timothy, Sandy Moss, the birth mother, was there. "I think it was probably the hardest thing I've ever had to do. Greg was crying, I was crying, she was crying. Everyone was very upset. And it was such a happy moment, but it was very, very, very sad." Charlotte says it is like two women in love with the same man: there are two women in love with the same baby. Through adoption, however, one woman gives the responsibility of mothering to the other. It is a deliberate decision.

How can the birth mother be valued in a way that does not demean her and reduce her to just a vessel to produce a child? And how can the adopting mother be valued in a way that gives her entitlement to call the child *my baby*? Charlotte was at the birth, and when Betsy was born, Rosie Smith, the birth mother, whispered, "I want to be the first to hold the baby." After a moment or two of holding her baby, Rosie said to her Betsy, "Now you go to your mother." "I just folded," says Charlotte. "It was the first time I was called a mother." Rosie gave Charlotte entitlement to be a mother. No one was demeaned or forgotten. This story is not a fiction. The birth of a child is also the birth of a mother, or—more accurately in the case of adoption— two mothers. Both women, as mothers, are present. They acknowledge each other's motherhood.

A Place to Belong

Through open adoption the birth mothers are given the opportunity and responsibility to choose the parents and the home for their child. The birth mother is given a number of files to read, which contain a copy of the home study report and a letter from the adopting parents. There may also be a picture of the parents and the home. The adopting parents talk about this process—where the birth mother chooses the mother and father for her child—as *being matched*. The birth mothers are not trying to be matched, that is, to find adopting parents who are like them. Rather, they are looking to find adopting parents that fit their picture of the right place for their child. The right match seems like a dream of finding the *if only* family: "This is the home I would want for my child if only I had what it takes to make my dream come true." Sometimes—as we have heard from both the adopting mother, Barbara, and the placing mother, Pauline—once the child is born, in spite of having found the adopting parents, the birth mothers think of ways to provide that home themselves.

The right place for the child may be with a woman who cannot have babies, or it may be a home with two parents, stability, and financial security. It may be where there is the possibility of a bike or music lessons—things that make sure "the child would not want for anything." Mary Sebastian says she wants to find parents who "can't have kids at all. Not a younger couple. Don't have to be rich or anything. Just happy." In many ways, instead of matching, one notices that the birth mothers are very different from the adopting mothers. Birth mothers are often young, have not finished their education, have no job, no home, and are not ready to care for a child. A good match for the birth mother seems to be finding the mother (or the parents) that will give her child exactly what she herself wishes she could give—whatever the image of that perfect home is.

Lorrie Newton. Responsible choice

"I had a little picture in my head. The white picket fence picture. But after a while I sort of realized that wasn't the way it was for me. And if I kept the baby I felt I would be being selfish. Because I don't have anything to offer a child. I think it would be too hard, because I'd have to work two, three jobs and never see the child, which isn't fair. And being raised in daycare is not my idea of a family. So I just thought it would be better off. I do have a lot to offer a child but not . . . I don't feel it's enough. I had a totally unstable environment. It was awful. I don't speak with my mother. She didn't do a fine job and that's probably one of the biggest reasons why I'm giving it up, because of the way I was raised by her. I don't want to turn into that kind of parent. She was never around, she was drunk all the time, and I'm scared that I could turn into that. I never knew my dad. And that bugged me, and it was worse on my brother. I think it's worse on a boy, not to have a father. I was pretty resilient. Nothing really bothered me when I was a kid, but my brother was really traumatized, I guess, by not having the male figure. He grew up kind of screwed up because of it.

"We [Lorrie and the birth father] got the files of seven couples the first time. We picked one couple out of there. And then the social worker gave us six the second time, and we picked two out of there. So out of thirteen couples we got three, and one of them was off the list. It took about two weeks—we decided on the one. I guess they called me Monday night and said, 'Do you want to meet?' And I said, 'Sure.' So we went out last night, the four of us, and talked and stuff.

"I have the option if I want the baby to room in with me while I'm in the hospital. And I figure, as long as I can handle it, without getting too attached, then I'll keep the baby with me. I'd like to be with him as much as possible before—I guess maybe three days at the most. It really won't be that much. Still, a lot of bonding can happen. I don't know if I'll be able to handle it that long. I want to spend a little time anyway. Actually we're going to be able to meet the child as well. But we don't know how we're going to arrange it yet. Maybe just sneak in as friends of the family or something. And the kid won't know who we are at first, for the first probably ten years or something. We'll be around probably once a year or so. Just to say hi. Because I want to be able to see the child. I think I'd go crazy if I couldn't. Want to know what he's up to, what he looks like, how he moves. Everything. That's why I went through open adoption, because through the government they just take the kid and you never see him again. I don't think I could handle that. That's not what I want at all. That's why at first I said I couldn't give up my baby, but this way they—you know, the people that we picked—said, 'We understand if you want a lot of pictures.' I said 'Great.' I want as much contact as is okay. I don't want to interfere in their lives or the way they're raising the child. But I want to know how the baby's changing and I want to know the different looks the kid has.

"I'm so fascinated by pregnancy. I'm just sitting here and saying it over and over, 'Wow, is it ever great.' 'Cause it is. The most incredible feelings. It makes me . . . like, my granny said, 'When the baby starts to kick a lot, you're going to get really uptight, and it's going to bug you and stuff.' And I said, 'It doesn't bug me at all. I smile all the time.' Every time it kicks, I'm like, whoo-hoo. This is neat. And I get all my friends, 'Feel this!' It doesn't bother me at all, because I'm just so happy about it. But then I feel the guilt feelings too—about the baby, giving up the baby. Sometimes when the baby kicks it makes me cry, because I feel so attached and then I know I'm not going to be able to keep it. But my mind's got to be in control, because this could ruin the kid's life, you know. Well, not ruin it, but it will probably have a lot more chances for things in life if he has the two-parent family and security. That's why I wanted to make my decision before I really talked to anyone, 'cause I didn't want anyone trying to influence me at all. I just wanted to do what I thought was best. And actually I was really torn up and I had really bad stress for a while. I was getting migraines. I think it was the stress of not knowing what I was doing. So once I decided to give up the baby I felt a lot better.

"I'm trying to imagine it, but I can't even imagine how I'm going to feel after. Because I might just snap back and say, 'Okay, I've done the right thing.' I still get to see my child. I'm still going to know where the child is and how the health is, and it's okay. Or else I might go the other way and just flip right out and say, 'I want my kid.' So, it's hard to tell which way. But usually I'm pretty strong and I feel I've done the right thing, I should be okay with it. I figure it is the responsible choice."

The women who place their babies want their children to have a place where they will belong. Often this means that the children will have something that their birth mothers did not have themselves. Lorrie did not have a sense of belonging and care from her mother and wants a different home for her child.

As the woman places her child with the adopting mother, the ownership of the child is transferred from one woman to another. Or is it? In adoption questions of ownership of the child come to light in vivid color. It seems that giving a child a home, a place to belong, gets confused with the notion of ownership. We often use the language of ownership when we talk of children: This is *my* child. We seem to think we own children by being responsible for their everyday activities, providing food, clothing, education, and other important life needs.

A few years ago, the parents of an infant, K'aila, who had a disease of the liver that resulted in death, decided against a liver transplant for their baby (Paulette 1993). When K'aila was three months old, he was diagnosed with a terminal liver disease for which the only possible solution was a liver transplant. His parents considered all the options for treatment—consulting medical texts and experts, reflecting on their cultural and spiritual traditions and values—in their decision against the transplant. The doctor recommending the transplant reported the family to the social welfare department. Following a long and difficult legal process, the judge ruled in favor of the parents. At eleven months of age, K'aila died at home in the arms of his family. To support his decision to report the parents to the child welfare department, the physician claimed that parents are not owners but stewards, and that in this case society must make the decision. The societal collective must decide about ownership or stewardship of the child—it can be a matter of life or death. When we think of ownership or stewardship of the child, we must remember that the child is society's child in very real ways. In one sense, *my* child is everyone's child.

To own (from the Indo-European root *eik*, meaning to possess) is very different from being a steward (which derives from the Indo-European *wer*, meaning to watch over) (Morris 1975). But what does it mean to be a steward of a child? How can one take responsibility for a child without taking on the child as a possession? Is there a way of conceiving of one's own child without an attitude of possessiveness? Can we think of *my child* instead of *my* child? The need to consider the question of ownership becomes clearer when we think of adoption. If we could think of the responsibility of the child as ours rather than believing the individual child to be ours, we might be more attentive to the interests of all—the child, the birth mother, and the adopting mother. It is the humanity of the child that calls us to think about the best place for the child, and it is the humanity of society that calls us to respect the experience of the two mothers involved.

The recent custodial fights between birth parent(s) and adopting parents show the great difficulties in treating children as possessions, as property that *belongs* to us. We seem to feel we own children by the names we give them. Will she be Anna or will she be Jessica? Will he be Jordan or will he be David? In everyone's eyes the public use of the name David Tearoe (the baby's adoptive name) severs his connection with his mother, Teena Sawan, who had named the boy Jordan (Tanner 1993). When Allison Decker talks of Cindy, the daughter whom she placed through government adoption services (closed adoption) three days after birth, she knows that Cindy may not be using that name anymore. Likely she has been given a different name by the adopting parents. This process of renaming the child is meant—unintentionally perhaps—to erase the reality of the birth mother and the baby's connection to her. What if the naming, the gift of giving a name, belonged to the birth mother? What if the name were understood as the blessing the birth mother bestows on the child—a blessing that maintains the continuity of past experiences and relationships (Roberts and Robie 1981)? Adopting parents are told that it is a nice gesture to the birth mother to involve her in choosing a name. Would this "nice gesture" be given more status and value if giving the name were seen as recognition that children are not owned, and that parenting can be shared in such a way that no one loses and everyone gains? Would this assist in the ongoing acknowledgment that the gift of a child is a gift that cannot be given away?

Rosie Smith cried all night after she placed her baby in the adopting mother's arms. She needed to put tea bags on her eyes to reduce the swelling. When John Elias, the adopting father, heard this, he said, "We can't take her child." He is right, they cannot. But they can take responsibility for this child and become her parents—to love, to watch over, to be with the child. And they have. But they do not own the child, nor does her birth mother. In order to help acknowledge the transfer of responsibility from birth mother to adopting parents, John prepared a ritual which took place before he and Charlotte took the baby home. This ritual, with two candles lit to symbolize the birth mother and the nurturing mother, illustrates the notion that responsibility rather than ownership is the issue here. This ritual helped Rosie give her baby a home, a place to belong, with Charlotte and John, and helped Charlotte accept the entitlement of *mother* from Rosie. Rituals, like this one, have nothing to do with ownership. They have to do with the awe and wonder of the child, with what it means to be a mother or a father, with belonging.

A Way to Belong

Adopting mothers take the question of belonging in a different direction. How can they belong in society without a child? In the past women almost took having children for granted. Many women, if not most, expected to be mothers some day—it was expected of them. Now the life journey of women does not necessarily take them to motherhood. They do have a choice. Even if they do not choose pregnancy, there is greater possibility that they will or will not choose mothering. Many women still long for a child in their lives. They may feel like Joan Bell, who says that she always thought it was part of her life plan and when it did not happen she was saddened. They may feel like Jennifer Black, who thought life would pass her by if she and her husband did not have a child. They may, like Karin Perry, feel that having a child gives them freedom to get on with their life—untying some knots that hold them back from getting at things.

The words *belonging* (from Middle English, *belongen*, to thoroughly suit) and *longing* (from Middle English *longian*, meaning to yearn for) are tied together in relation to children. With a child in their arms, women who yearn for a child feel that they have a place. They belong, they are no longer on the outside; people talk to them at the store, and they can talk more easily with other women. The red BLOCK PARENT sign in the window of their home and the car seat securely fastened in the backseat of their car are brilliant symbols of their success. These symbols become warm reminders to these mothers that they finally belong. It may seem that these women do not feel complete in themselves, that they live through their children. Karin, however, suggests that fulfilling her desire to have a child in life frees her to be more who she already is.

Karin Perry. A bundle of knots untied

"The instant I held Emily, I felt recognition. She felt just right in my arms. She stared up at me and I stared back at her. We were definitely bonded from that instant. It was really wonderful." This is the day of my last discussion with Karin. Emily, the lovely brown-eyed, auburn-haired baby, is sleeping peacefully in the room next to her parents—the room where, for so long, the ironing board was kept. Her mother, Karin, says that finally the bundle of knots that tied up her energy is being untied. Karin says, "Maybe quite a large part of my energies were tied up, were focused inwardly, and now that knot has been untied and the energy is free to be used in interacting with people." In some ways, she expects to be able to do her work better, with more maturity and confidence, making her more influential, more focused and efficient.

"I think that the whole process has had an effect of opening me up more to other people and just generally being more open about my own feelings and more ready to accept friendship or to deepen friendship with other people. I remember I talked about getting to know the women in the IVF [in vitro fertilization] program quite well—I mean, you talk very frankly with them while waiting for these different tests and things. You talk about adoption especially. The whole process of having to really tell all and really think your way through everything affects one. I've always thought it's the most fundamental thing in life—being a parent. It's the one thing that makes us all carry on from generation to generation. It is the most important thing you can do. The whole process of thinking about it and writing about it and telling people about it over and over again as you do in talking to social workers and so on, and even talking to you, Vangie, just kind of opens you up. It makes you realize what you think about things—kind of gets the kinks out. I don't know if it happens to most mothers, maybe it does, maybe it doesn't. I mean, a lot of women become mothers just sort of without ever thinking about it much."

Karin married Gil when she was young, just twenty. Having a family was always, from the earliest age, something that was percolating, but not until she was twenty-nine did it take on steam. It may be that her infertility was a problem all along, which makes Karin wonder if all those birth control pills and diaphragms were a waste of money! During those years Karin was going to university, and is now reasonably established in her career.

She did not tell anyone at work that she was both planning to adopt and entering a program of in vitro fertilization. When it was time to go for the ten-day period of monitoring with blood tests and ultrasound so the fertilized embryos could be transferred into her uterus, people at work thought she had gone on a holiday to the mountains. She thought her colleagues might think she was not committed to her job, even though she thoroughly enjoyed it and spent long hours at it. She wanted them to think of her as a potential administrator, not a potential mother. It was some holiday! She made three visits daily to the hospital, where ten mature eggs were retrieved through pinholes in her vagina. These eggs were then fertilized by Gil's sperm in a petri dish. Six eggs were fertilized and three were reintroduced into her uterus. This trip cost them $5,000 plus the hotel room, some of which they hope to recover through insurance. The waiting was the hardest—waiting to find out if she was pregnant.

Her period started the day before the scheduled pregnancy test.

It was time to move, again, to adoption. "Adoption was there in your mind, every day, always there on the back burner. If only I could speed up the process of getting a baby. Whatever it takes. I don't think I'm incredibly committed to the idea that it need be *our own* baby. I just want one. But there are 180 couples on the waiting list."

Emily arrived suddenly. They were matched with young birth parents—eighteen and twenty. If the girl's family had been neighbors, they would have been good friends. The day the baby girl was born, Karin just couldn't stay home. Although she knew that she could not see the baby until the next day, Karin wanted to drive that night, so that she could be closer to the baby. She needed to go. This was not just an ordinary evening! "Erica and Bob, the birth parents, had arranged to be at the hospital by themselves that last day. We just met and talked with them for a few minutes and took some photos. They were both really good. Bob was really gentle with the baby. I could see that some day he will be a really good father. He was feeding Emily when we came in. He dressed her up in this sort of going-away outfit. It was really sweet. Erica was in the bathroom getting ready for the photos (a typical teenager). There wasn't really much to say. They showed us everything they had ready for her. Different relatives had given her little things. Erica's grandmother had made a lovely little yellow sweater and cap and there was another hand-knit thing, quite a few things, as well as the locket with pictures of Erica and Bob. All in a decorated box.

The belonging that is released in Karin is not the belonging of possession, but a belonging that she is a part of and in. "I take part in, am intimately involved with, a reality greater than myself, whether it is a love relationship, a community, a religion or the whole universe" (Capra and Steindl-Rast 1991: 14). Having a child, loving a child makes one find one's place, be at home in a community of others, family, friends—even the larger community of animals and trees. To belong as a mother is not to live through one's children, but to live more fully in oneself.

In adoption the sense of belonging takes another important twist, heard in Jennifer's poignant words, "I don't like to look eighteen years down the road and say the worst part is when they decide to go to their birth parent. I don't have any control over that. And if they decided to do that, well . . . I'll drive them." These words show a commitment to the child's need to belong, to find his or her own place, even if it is painful for the mother. Any child who is adopted has the legacy of another mother, other grandparents, other brothers and sisters. Where does this child belong? Can this child belong in both families? Jennifer's heartrending "I'll drive them" shows the ongoing adopting mother's reality: the birth mother is always present, to the child and to the mother. The birth mother ties the child to his or her roots.

Who is family? Karin talks of Emily's birth grandparents as Emily's grandparents. She says she almost wishes the birth mother, Erica, would keep in touch a bit more. She says, "Everyone that we have met in the birth family, from both sides of the birth family, are a fine family, and I think it can only benefit Emily to know them better. We are not at all worried about any concept like, she won't really be our child if we have to share her. I mean, it's good for children to have lots of people loving them." "People do not own each other and no matter how many people you love, there is still enough love for more" (Ryan 1990: 45).

Karin raises what she sees as a problem in maintaining connections with the birth mother. She says, "If Emily's birth background had been a negative one, like if her birth mother had been a street prostitute or something, then I would be anxious to protect her from seeing too much of that." The troubled background of the birth mother (or parents) is a factor that adoptive parents think about. In placing her child for adoption, the birth mother is moving from a difficult situation to offer her child the best possible life, a life she cannot provide herself. Can this be seen as a positive outcome from a difficult life circumstance? Does the placing of a child by the birth mother change what might be seen as a negative story to a positive one? Perhaps the judgment itself is to be questioned. If one is doing the very best that one can, is there such a thing as failure?

Adoption is for the child, and keeping in touch with the child's roots helps foster the child's sense of belonging—to the adopted family and to the birth family. The struggle experienced in open adoption is felt in Nel's words, "There's such a closeness between us, but you can't be too close. It's so hard, so hard. I'm probably more scared just out of my own insecurity, I'm afraid that he is not going to love me as much as he loves *her*, or something totally ridiculous like that. And in other ways I want her to come, I want her to see him and I want her to see us, and a very very small part of me wishes that she could be part of our family. Because she's given us so much and she's such a nice person. In one way I have a lot of love for her, and in another way I have a lot of fear." Here, again, love and fear are the experience of the mother. The adoptive mother loves her child and the child's mother, but she fears that the child will choose the birth mother in the end. "We like each other and I think that's the hardest part now, because I like her and she likes us, but I cannot have her in my life on a regular basis, you know!" says Nel.

It seems that birth mothers are looking for the right place, the right home for their child. They are giving the child a family, a family that will include themselves in some capacity. "There's a picture of him on my dresser," says Sally Corbett about the boy she placed for adoption. "And he looks *exactly* like me. Like, if I just pulled all my hair back, he would look exactly like me. People look at him and they say, 'do you have a little brother?' I say, 'no' and they go, 'who is that?' I say, 'oh, it's just a friend's baby.' And they say, 'well, geez, he looks an awful lot like you,' and I say, 'that's what everybody says.' " Who is family in open adoption? Is the birth mother just a friend of the family? Or is the birth mother *family*?

Gwen Reid. A friend among friends

The sputtering and choking of baby James provides a vivid backdrop for the discussion of how he came to be Gwen and Michael's child. He has bronchitis, and if the new medication does not improve him by the next day, his mother will take him to the hospital. Gwen and Michael talk about how having James has moved them from the "me, me, me" life of single people to the "us" of concern for another. It took more than marriage for Gwen and Michael—the move to the sense of *us* needed a child.

The birth mother had been at their home a couple of times—first to see how they lived and then to celebrate the baptism. At the baptism guests did not know that the woman holding and feeding the child was more than a friend among the friends and family who surrounded the baby and his parents. The birth mother fed her baby as his adoptive parents busied themselves with the celebration of this baby as a member of their family.

Before the birth of James, the birth mother, Fiona, came with three pages full of questions, as she still hadn't made her final choice of the adopting parents. "We knew that she had some serious interest, and she had serious concerns about her child's welfare." Gwen says, "You have to watch what you're saying, and hope everything you are saying is what she wanted to hear. I was really careful. I didn't want to seem forceful, I didn't want to seem overeager, but I did want to seem eager, because I was eager. If I didn't seem eager enough, she'd have thought that we don't want the child. I wanted to seem concerned for her, you know, as obviously I was, but you feel. . . ."

The birth parents had discussed marriage, but Fiona did not want marriage and the birth father, Lance, could not look after the child by himself. The birth parents met the adopting parents and there seemed to be a mutual checking, and mutual approval. When the baby was born, Gwen and Michael raced down to the hospital, hurried up to the room and walked in—hesitantly. There they found Lance sitting in the chair rocker, holding his baby, and Fiona sitting in the bed. Lance got up, came toward them, and handed Michael the baby. Michael held the baby for about three hours. "They coached us on feeding—'his next feeding is eight and nine, but you should have a bath demonstration and you can feed him after that, then you should be back here.' " Fiona decided what we were to do. It was nerve-racking at first, because you know you're holding this baby and you're saying it's ours, it's ours, it's ours, but maybe it's not ours. Something can always happen. This is their baby and they are watching us and what we do. 'I'm not holding it right.' 'Should I, you know, look more confident with it?' 'Should I leave them alone?' 'Do they need time to themselves?' She kept saying 'no.'

"We met her mother and sister and one of the relatives and the neighbor, and they came to visit her at the hospital. We left the hospital with James at the same time as they did, like the nurse walked off with us, the five of us. They left while we got him arranged in the car seat. That was a very emotional time for the father, Lance—really, really emotional. I guess Fiona had accepted it and been able to come to terms more readily with it. Lance was really emotionally shaken. It was a couple of days later, and he called up on his way back home. He wanted to see where we lived, and he dropped by and gave us pictures of us in the hospital, of us holding him, of them holding him, of the five of us together. We got on very well with the father, maybe it was because of a similar background—both had a similar background—so we could relate to him. There's a very good match.

It is Michael who describes their experience of having this baby. "It is something . . . something that we could not have, and yet now we have. We can't put a finger on it. It is just total awe. There's nothing in this world that would compare to a little baby. There's no gift as great. Somebody gave us their child. When you are single you live day to day, easygoing, happy-go-lucky, if my time was up tomorrow, so be it. Now with a baby you want to see him grow up, see his children, you want to mold him. It is harder to leave this life when you have a baby."

The adopting parents often comment that people look for family resemblances in the baby. This ties families together. "A friend of mine commented that Tim [their adopted son] has a cowlick. And it's on exactly the same side as Greg's," says Nel. But Nel is less concerned that he looks like family—she just wants him to feel comfortable. Yet Nel's mother feels differently. Nel's mother and father, in announcing the arrival of the new baby, do not want to say anything about the adoption. "He's ours," they say, "and you don't need to tell anybody." Sally, a birth mother, with her mother and other relatives got to know the adopting parents very well. Karin, an adopting mother, feels that the birth mother's family could be good friends—special friends that need special care. The question that comes up with both mothers is, "How to be close and not too close?" How can the adoption be open and yet not too open? How can the birth mother be a part of her child's life without interfering in that life? Is the birth mother called a special friend, a favorite auntie, or just a friend of the family? How can the child feel that he or she belongs *in* the family without belonging *to*—that is, being owned by—the family?

The gift of a baby is a responsibility that moves one from a self-centered notion of life to a focus beyond one's self. Through the birth mother's decision, the adopting mother is given the gift of a lifetime and beyond. For the adopting mother and father, the gift of a child requires a decision of "Yes, I will accept this child, I will be responsible for, provide for, and take this child as my child." It is a decision of the heart and the mind. The birth mother's responsibility seems the opposite. The birth mother has to say "no" with her mind; her body has already said "yes" to the child, and the child already belongs, is tied to her. Her heart and her mind have to say "no" for the sake of the child, and for her own sake.

Adopting mothers and birth mothers are forging new extended families. These families include grandparents, aunts, and uncles that come from both birth and adopting families. These new relationships have to be worked out. Sometimes the birth mother is almost like a daughter to the adopting mother, or the birth grandmother is the child's only grandmother. Emily's birth grandparents visit regularly, and the adopting parents are happy that they do. James's birth father is very much like the adopting father. Both of these families love the child. The challenge of open adoptions is to forge new relationships between the two families of the child, the birth family and the adopting family. To hold deep and lifelong love for the child as central, these families have to forge a new reality, where commitment to the child is a way of belonging and not of ownership.

In the next chapter I will discuss the experience of teens in their move to motherhood. The emphasis will be on the sense of support these women need and get from the community and from their own mothers. All mothers need support. The teen mothers bring this need to full awareness.

NOTE

1. Susan James is acknowledged for writing the first version of Pauline's story.

4

Teen Mothers

Many times during my conversations with pregnant teenage women I was struck by both their strength and their vulnerability. There were times when they seemed to be little girls needing my support and protection—I wanted to take them home with me. There were other times when they seemed to be strong, determined women—I felt enormous respect for their courage and their honesty of expression. It may be that both fragile vulnerability and enormous strength characterize these teenage mothers who, while children themselves, choose to raise their own children. In some ways the teen mothers show, in stark nakedness, what it means to be a mother. They show the strength and the vulnerability that all women who mother experience. Throughout this chapter I refer to these girl women as teen mothers to show my acknowledgment of them as growing from the young girls they are to the strong women they also are.

Teen mothers often talk about growing up with their children. They see this as a strength, and so do I, because, being young, these teen mothers have great potential for change and growth while being intertwined with the growth and care of their children. The teen mother, through the experiences and practices of mothering, is able to "introduce significance, meaning, identity, and a future within the possibilities and constraints of her immediate situation and the wider social understandings of what it is to be a woman and a mother," says Lee SmithBattle (1994: 159). It is not that the teen mother remakes herself into a mother, but mothering remakes her, claims SmithBattle, for "the experience of loving and being loved by a child offers a corrective experience that contrasts with her own painful and troubled past" (1994: 151). Not all teenage mothers have what SmithBattle refers to as a troubled past, but it does seem that teen mothers do experience a time of confusion, turmoil, and uncertainty. The use of the word "corrective" shows the attitude of judgment that is often associated with teen mothers. A stronger understanding of this word may be what the mothers themselves experience—a transformation that moves them to think about others as well as themselves. Having *a child on her mind* changes how the teen mother sees herself and her world.

There is no doubt that teen mothers desire to be good mothers. They want to be the best mothers and provide the best for their children, as we hear from Celine Merrill: "I want the best for my child, I want to give my child a better life than what I had." And while these teen mothers have a strong desire to do the right thing for their child, they have desires for themselves as well. They want to finish high school, to become pediatricians, writers, psychologists, nurses, or childcare workers. Ruth-Ann Stapleton says, "I want to have everything. I want to have a good education and I don't want to be involved in violence and alcohol." They desire the same as other mothers in wanting the best for their children and themselves. But desire may not be enough. These mothers, just like all mothers, cannot do it alone. How can we, the community, support teen mothers to be the very best mothers they can be?

In this chapter I share the words and stories of a small group of teen mothers about their experiences during the last weeks of pregnancy and the early weeks of childcare. Their words and stories show us their lives, tell *the* story of how these teens move to motherhood. Barry Lopez believes that "stories—fiction and non-fiction—offer us a way to re-imagine our lives" (1995:39). These stories offer a way to reimagine the lives of these young women. We can step away from their stories with a renewed sense of the potential of teen mothers, with new respect for their experience. Only if we recognize and appreciate their experience, what they go through, can we support them in imagining their lives, to make their dreams come true for their babies and themselves.

Mothers are born by bringing children into their lives. Mothers are not simply born by the bodily act of giving birth to a baby, important as that is for them. Rather, women are born into mothering through the culture in which they live. Teen mothers frequently say that they are mothers just like other mothers. Celine clearly states, "I'm capable of being a mother just as well as a thirty-year-old is, you know. I'm probably more responsible than a lot of adults out there." There is, however, a community expectation that one should not become a mother until some things are in place—completed education, financial stability, marriage, and so on. There is a general sense, now, that the teen years are not the best time to have children. It is felt that these women are just too young, too inexperienced, and too unstable. Teen pregnancy gets special attention. One example of such attention is the *People* magazine's Special Report (Gleick et al. 1994) titled "Babies Who Have Babies," which describes the cycle of hardship and privation perpetuated by teen pregnancy. Often pregnancy for a single teen mother is seen as a dilemma that has no easy solution—in fact no solution at all. Whatever these young women decide to do about their pregnancy (abortion, placement, or keeping), their choices pose dilemmas (Farber 1991). If one thinks about teen pregnancy as a societal problem, then one may be able to think about solutions, such as better education, decreasing poverty, or increasing options for work to make a living. But once a particular teen becomes pregnant, she is not a problem that can be solved; rather, she has to live with her choice in the best way possible. Whatever decision she makes about her pregnancy, she will remember her experience and feel the repercussions, challenges, and joys of it for the rest of her life.

When teen mothers are seen as a social problem they are immediately stigmatized: "What should we do about the problem of teen pregnancy?" When teen mothers say that they are the same as other mothers, in that they can physically give birth like other women, they are correct. In fact, they may have an easier time. In current Western culture, however, with its social attitudes against teen pregnancy, the experience of teen pregnancy, birth, and care of the child is very different than it is for older, married mothers. It seems that teen mothers have many strikes against them—they are often single, poor, still in school, living with their parents, and considered irresponsible. Yet, if we attempt to understand the individual experiences of the teen mothers who keep their babies, listen to their stories, and love them, we may think of useful ways to support them in this new responsibility of mothering.

Teen mothers do talk about the pain of labor and birth, yet it is not the bodily pain that they focus on. Rather, it is the pain of being censored by everyone. Teen mothers have to prove themselves capable and responsible, because they are not expected or assumed to be responsible. Yet, their sense of responsibility is an overriding theme in this chapter. Teen mothers take on responsibility for many things—their babies, their relationships, their schooling, their finances, and even finding the right place to live.

Most of the conversations with teen women in this study took place at school, while some, especially after the birth of their baby, occurred in their homes. Jasmine Jonson (fifteen years old), Holly Radcliff (eighteen), Rachel O'Donnell (seventeen), Celine Merrill (sixteen), Carole Benson (seventeen), Michelle Freeman (seventeen), Ruth-Ann Stapleton (fifteen), and Jesse Abbott (sixteen) speak about their experiences. They do not speak with one voice, for they have different experiences. Nor do they speak for all teen mothers. These women speak for themselves. By understanding more about the particularities of the experiences of teen mothers, we can understand more about what teen mothers desire and what they need.

The first focus of attention for teens, once pregnancy is realized, is to make a decision about what to do. Although the final choice is up to the teen herself, she almost always makes it with assistance from others. Relationships with others are important for her—relations with the father of the child, her family, friends, and people within the community where she lives. School, too, is an important consideration.

THE DECISION TO KEEP

It's hard to accept. There's no easy way out of being pregnant. You have to think about abortion, you have to think about adoption, you have to think about keeping. And it's just really hard because there's no easy way out. It's the hardest decision you can make in your life. (Carole Benson)

At seventeen, Carole Benson knows what it is like to grow up fast. It means, first and foremost, making decisions of enormous impact. Making decisions to give birth and to nurture are not easy. One has to decide whether or not to have an abortion. One has to decide whether or not to place the child for adoption. These are huge decisions with huge consequences. Each possibility is tested, tried out, and tried on. What will it mean for me to keep this child? How will my family react? How will my friends respond? What about the father? Is he here for me and the child? Do I want him to be here? Carole tells us what it is like for her. She, like the others, realizes that this decision is probably the most important one she'll ever make. Many teen pregnancies do end in abortion. Some teen mothers place their babies for adoption, and an increasing number keep their children to raise themselves. They do have a choice and they do struggle with it.

Carole Benson. No easy way out

Like many of the sexually active teens, Carole was not using any birth control. "Well, it just never occurred to me that I could get pregnant, so I didn't. I was on the pill, but I stopped taking it for some reason or other. Not because I wanted to get pregnant. I think I just forgot."

The baby's father was a few years older and Carole calls him a real jerk. "He's immature. And he's irresponsible. I didn't like the way he told me what to do all the time, saying, 'You do this or I'll take the baby away from you' and stuff like that. So I just got rid of him. He's a bum. I went through rough morning sickness. I had morning sickness every single day, for a long time. And it was just really bad, because I was missing school—weeks at a time. I'd go to school and I'd have to come home because I'd be throwing up. And he didn't really care, didn't seem to care. I was always chasing after him, you know, looking for sympathy and stuff. And he never really gave me any, so I just said, 'Forget it.' Didn't need that any more.

"I went through a really rough time in my life. I got involved with a lot of undesirables, I guess you could call them. I wasn't going to the doctor for a pregnancy test—just a general check-up. When he said I was pregnant I was shocked. I was really scared to tell my mum, so I phoned her. I told her over the phone. And I didn't go home that night. And when I went home the next day we talked about it and my mum cried. And it made me feel so bad. My dad cried too. It made me grow up. And my mum, she even said that I've changed a lot. I'm back to my normal self. There was three years, when I turned fifteen, things just went downhill. I ran away from home on my fifteenth birthday. I've always wanted to go to college, but I didn't know what I wanted to be. I stopped caring about my schoolwork for a long time, and I'm supposed to graduate this year. But I won't. I can't graduate.

"People look at you. I notice that people stare at pregnant women. But they look at me with a sort of look of disgust on their face. Especially older people, senior citizens, you know, look at you kind of funny. And you think, 'Well, how do you think you got here? I mean, your mum was probably the same age as me when she was pregnant with you!' When I used to see teenagers pregnant I used to think, 'Oh look at that!' Now, it's different. And when people aren't pregnant, your friends and stuff, they always say, 'Well, you should keep the baby, it'll be so cute.' But they don't realize how hard it is to keep a baby. And they don't realize . . . I think, sure, they'll come over and see the baby, and if it starts crying, give it back to mum, you know. They're not here overnight for the two o'clock feedings, and the diaper changes, and when the baby gets sick and is spitting up, and it won't stop crying and stuff. They don't know how hard it is. They don't realize the responsibility. So they have a biased opinion.

"It was just a decision I had to make on my own."

Carole is living at home and has support from both her father and mother. Her baby Jeremy sleeps in her room. "There were a couple of nights when I just cried, because he won't go to sleep and he'd just cry. I didn't know what to do with him. Like he'd just cry and he'd cry and I'd calm him down. He would calm down, then he'd wake up again and he'd cry. I didn't know what to do with him any more. My mom came into my room after four. He had screamed from one o'clock. She took him. She said, 'Goodnight.' She turned off my light and left with him. I was just exhausted. I was crying."

In talking with Carole and the other teen mothers, at times it seemed to me as if they made the decision without really making a decision, that is, as if they did not do anything at all—their decision was made. Since they did not do anything, the child remained with them. It was like getting pregnant—they did not decide, they just lived as if pregnancy could not happen to them. They had birth control pills but did not take them. Some teens said that they did not get pregnant on purpose, yet did nothing to prevent pregnancy—they did not think about the consequences of their sexual activity. They just went along as if nothing would happen.

Research on the sociodemographic and biographic characteristics of teen mothers who choose childrearing versus adoption indicates that teen mothers who choose childrearing tend to have lower socioeconomic status and lower educational aspirations, come from families with a higher incidence of teen pregnancy, and say that they cannot emotionally handle the thought of adoption (Resnick, Blum, Bose, Smith, and Toogood 1990). While research of that nature is interesting and useful in understanding the general picture of teen mothers and the choices they make, it tells nothing of the individual teen's experience: What it is like for her? How do her decisions affect her life? I attempt to show the experience of teen mothers, like Celine Merrill, who look to the future and "take it one step at a time."

Breaking the News

Many teens are reluctant to tell their parents, or others, about their pregnancy. Some keep it a secret for a while, and even when they do tell their parents, the pregnancy is often kept secret from the extended family. Michelle Freeman says that her dad said to her mother, "What are you doing telling everyone she's pregnant? You don't want people to know." Michelle says that at first she thought that her father would send her away some place "till I had the kid." Given the societal concern about teen pregnancy, the reaction of these parents is not unusual. It is expected. Teen pregnancy is often accompanied by anger, tears, sadness, rage, yelling, or "flipping out." No teen reported any happiness in breaking the news of her pregnancy to her parents. Pregnancy is seen negatively by every parent, for it diverts the expected path for their daughter—finishing school, getting a job, getting married, and so on. Families are disappointed and often worry about their daughter's future (Farber 1991). How different this reaction is from how parents usually react when an older, married, daughter is going to have a baby!

For many pregnant teens the possibility of having an abortion is suggested by parents, and is often the first response to the pregnancy. For others, the possibility of adoption is raised as the best way to respond. But the teen mothers in this study chose—for many reasons, such as "did not believe in abortion," or "could not imagine giving the baby away"—to raise their child themselves. Michelle's words show how the teen mother experiences her decision differently than others, even the baby's father. Michelle says that while her boyfriend talks of giving the baby up for adoption, she is having a bodily experience of the baby inside her. She says, "like, all the time he's saying this the kid's sitting there kicking me in the stomach. I couldn't, I couldn't handle it, like, to give it up to perfect strangers." We see again that the decision to have a child—and the decision about what to do about an unwanted pregnancy—is not just rational, but is experienced in the body. It is not a simple, firm, final decision. It is rather more like *coming to* a decision. Decision-making about whether or not to have and keep a baby is complex (Farber 1991) and is influenced by values, dreams, and imagination.

Once the decision to keep the child themselves is made, the teens seek support and acceptance of that decision (Farber 1991). All the teen mothers in this study, except for Celine, gained the support of their families (especially their mothers) during the pregnancy and after the birth. In fact, it seems that in the end parents and siblings often become excited and happy about the birth of the baby. Celine was the only teen mother who had no immediate family support during her baby's birth and for a few months after the birth. In later correspondence, however, Celine informed me that she, too, had reconnected with her own mother and now has her full support.

Coming to a Decision

We wonder how the teen mother comes to making such a hard decision. What influences her choice to keep her baby? Teens are frequently perceived of as being unable to make responsible choices. Recall Jesse Abbott's experience when her child was hospitalized and she needed her own mother's signature for treatment of her baby (see chapter three). Do we think that teens are too self-centered? Too unrealistic? Just too young? Some of us may wonder if they can realistically decide to keep their child. Teen mothers do not have much time—less than nine months—to decide what to do. Does having a baby fill a need? Does it give them someone to love and to love them? Does it give a certain kind of prestige? Does it get attention? Some people think teens become mothers in order to gain independence from family or to qualify for welfare. The teens themselves wonder if they will be able to look after the baby and still attend school, have enough money, or have a life of their own.

One wonders, too, about influences like a recent advertisement for Joop Jeans (Hogarth 1995). This advertisement has a woman dressed in jeans holding a leash with a dog collar around a baby's neck. The ad reads: A CHILD IS THE ULTIMATE PET. In advertisements like this one women are portrayed as young, white, passive, vulnerable, and available. Their bodies are relentlessly used to sell products and ideas. What is the cumulative effect of these inaccurate portrayals of young women on their life choices and decisions? This ad combines jeans and sex—with the child as a possession, something to be valued or to give one value. But of course a child is not a pet, a prize, or a status symbol. We know that choosing whether to keep a baby or not is not the same as keeping or returning a pair of jeans that do not fit or are the wrong color. Yet we also know that advertisements affect us in ways not readily recognized. While many factors contribute to the decision to have and to keep a baby, one needs to attend to societal influences. It may be wise to explore the whole picture of influences—such as the advertisement cited above—that affect the decision, or the nondecision, of young women becoming pregnant and keeping their babies.

For pregnant teen mothers the decision about abortion is often the first consideration. Jasmine Jonson says, "My first plans were to abort it, because my mom told me, 'let's just forget about this, let's get out of here, and things will go back to normal,' and she never thought about the baby or anything. Then I went for an ultrasound and they told me how many weeks I was pregnant. Then I said 'forget it.' " Jasmine thought she would hate her mother forever if she complied with her mother's initial demand that she have an abortion. For Rachel O'Donnell, no matter what her mother told her, the "blob" in her belly was a baby, and she could not abort it. Although Celine easily decided against abortion, she did think about adoption. But then she talks of her vision of the family she would have with her boyfriend, William, for she says, "This is the person I want to be with for the rest of my life." She wants to give him a baby and expects him to give her the support she needs. For others the decision to keep the child is present all along—perhaps to replace some previously felt loss. The actual influences vary. Yet, for each there are strong reasons calling her to make the decision to keep the child. The process of deciding may not be any different than for an older woman who is faced with an unexpected and unwanted pregnancy. Yet, with teen mothers the options are faced openly and directly.

Going to a school for teen mothers made a difference for these women. At school they had a chance to discuss their options with other pregnant teens. For example, Jesse Abbott talked with other young women who had even fewer resources than she had and who had decided to keep their babies. This led Jesse to think, "If they can keep, so can I." Later, however, Jesse placed her son for adoption and thinks that she had a very unrealistic idea of what keeping the child would mean to her. Some teen mothers feel it is selfish to place a child, because it is like passing the responsibility on to someone else; others feel it is selfish to keep the child, because they would not be able to provide for the child. It is a lose-lose situation.

For many of the teen mothers it is not clear what they should do—but it is clear that they are the decision-makers. They talk to others about it, yet it is ultimately up to them. In all situations they need real, concrete support. With Celine, it is knowing that William wants this baby and would stay around to help her. With Rachel, it is having a mother to share an apartment with. With others, it means continuing to live at home. Teen mothers need the support of others: financial support from parents and social services; daily support from families and boyfriends; school support from administrators and institutions; and conversational support from other pregnant women and teen mothers. It is their decision whether or not they will keep the baby, but they cannot act on that decision alone. Just like all mothers, they need support.

Babies Are Cute

"Oh, it's a baby, how cute," is what Carole thinks her friends who do not have babies say. "I thought it would be fun to have a baby. Whenever you see a baby or you babysit, it's fun. You don't realize it is so much work," states Ruth-Ann Stapleton. Yes, babies are cute. Almost everyone agrees. Babies attract us. Yet, as Carole says, the notion that babies are cute does not reflect the reality of living with a baby. The idea that "babies are cute" plays down the extent of the responsibility, of the day-to-day, hour-to-hour work that these teen mothers do in caring for their babies. We, together with them, wonder whether the decision to keep is always the best one, or whether it is made thinking about all the nice things about babies, not realizing the difficult nights, the long days, and the hard work that the care of babies demands. Were the teen mothers caught, like many of their friends, in the idea that "babies are cute," without really understanding the reality of the baby crying all night, as Carole describes? Did these teens really know how much a baby would cost? Celine discusses the money needed to support her and her baby, both before and after the birth. Some of her figures seem unrealistic given economic realities. For example, Celine says that she will save her change (quarters and dollars), so as to provide a pocket of money for her child. The real costs involved in raising a child are not known. Before pregnancy teens do not generally think much about money, but once pregnant, finances become an important concern. Still, they think a five-dollar-an-hour wage is pretty good. They do not realize ahead of time that this wage may not be enough to provide all the things they want for themselves and their baby.

Celine's words show the misconceptions that she and others have about money. She says, "Like, I want to save money for other things as well. I don't want to have ratty furniture all the time. I'm going to try and buy some new furniture and stuff like that." She thinks about how to use the money that social welfare provides to help her set up her own apartment when she gets independent status. "Social services is going to give me about two thousand dollars. They're going to give me $225 for a crib and I'm not going to need $225 for a crib, I know that fact. At the most I'm going to need $150, so I'll have an extra $75 to spend. And I think I'll put that aside for furniture." When I ask Celine if she has any experience with money and budget she tells me about the paper delivery job that she had for a few years and about the accounting course she will take at school next year. Later, when I visit her at her apartment, she had some old and some new furniture. She still did not have enough money for a stroller. Celine and Will were planning to save to buy the stroller, which would give her a chance to get out of the apartment. They learned the economics of living with a baby only once they had the child in their life.

The decision-making about the baby comes during a time of intense drama in these young women's lives: young love, sexual explorations, school demands, separating from family, leaving home. For many, it is a time of intense personal turmoil, often a time when their comings and goings are outside of their parents' control and even—it seems—of their own control. In thinking back on the experience of making the decision, Holly Radcliff wonders, "Did I do the right thing?"

Holly Radcliff. I'm too young for this

"I told my mom first. Like she was just shocked. She told my dad. I should have told him, but I felt I needed my time to be able to tell him. When he found out he just flipped. He said, "You are having an abortion." He felt that the way to handle a problem is to get rid of it. I told him there was no way I would do that. Then he wanted me to place the baby once it's born."

Holly did not believe that she could ever become pregnant—something about an emergency surgery when she was aged two led her to this belief. "When I met Robert I went on the pill, and then I went off it. I wasn't doing it on purpose, like I wasn't doing it to get pregnant. I had been sexually active without having any birth control before and I just figured that I couldn't get pregnant, simple! Me and Robert had gone for two months without even having any birth control at all and nothing. I just wish I would've been on the pill. I don't know, in a way, I still feel I'm too young for this. I would have waited, you know, till me and Robert settled all of our problems, so that we were, like, not fighting any more."

Holly and Robert, who had split up, got reconciled when Holly discovered that she was pregnant. "I realized something's wrong here, so we both went to the doctor, and we've been together since. We realized that his mom was a single mom raising him, and he doesn't want that for our child at all, so he wants our child to have two parents."

Pregnancy was difficult for Holly. Severe backache led her to take leave from her job and stay in bed. "Because I'm so small the baby is finding it very hard to move around in there, and I couldn't even get out of bed. That's how bad the pain was. I couldn't go Christmas shopping or anything." But she says, "When I feel stress and tension, this baby does too. The baby kicks a lot. When me and Robert are yelling and arguing at each other, then this baby is like 'what the heck are you guys doing' kind of thing. When I feel stress or am upset or crying or whatever, this baby is like going 'mom, it's okay' kind of thing."

Holly's family slowly developed support for her decision to keep the baby. Her younger brother even became excited. Robert did not tell anybody in his family other than his mother about Holly's pregnancy. "His grandparents, aunts, uncles don't have a clue."

Holly found that her school friends could not accept her pregnancy. "I said, if you can't accept it, I don't need you right now." She switched to a special school and found far more support there. "I like coming here, because the girls that I know now have gone through what I've gone through and are going through what I'm going through."

"The baby's due five days after my nineteenth birthday. If it comes on my birthday, I'll just die. I want to be at home with my presents and my cake and my family, you know, I don't want to be in some hospital." Her son, Neil, was born two weeks early. Like her mother's and her grandmother's, Holly's labor was fast. Robert attended the birth. "It was funny because Robert said, 'I'm not watching. Forget it. That's gross.' Yet, he was down there the whole time. I'm just like 'get up here. You're my coach, not the doctor. Get up here.'"

Holly is responsible for Neil at night. He sleeps in her room. But she isn't sure that she really feels like a mother. "I'm not on my own. Like, I will feel like a mother when I move out and I have to do the dishes and the laundry all the time, but not really now, because I'm living at home with my parents. It's really hard. Like last Monday Robert didn't take him, 'cause we didn't have school, and I'm just like, 'Can you please take him?' My parents babysit a lot for me. It's like . . . my parents are babysitting and I hear him crying and I'm just like, 'are they going to go and get him, or am I supposed to get him, or what?' They're like, 'oh, go upstairs and do your homework,' but he's crying and everything, and I have to go downstairs and check on him.

"My boyfriend says, 'You're so boring now.' And I say, 'I'm sorry, there's nothing I can do. We stayed home on New Year's. What can I do, like go to the bar and look like a total idiot, like 'hi, I'm the only sober one in this place'? I didn't want to do anything like that. I should not be going out to the bar or doing this, doing that—things like what my friends from my other school are doing. That's the hardest part. Friday night I stay home. Saturday night I stay home. It's not like we used to be."

Mostly, Holly believes she made a good decision. "Just having Neil. He's mine and that's the best part. Sometimes I do think, you know, maybe it would have been better if I would have given him up for adoption. Would he be better right now? Of course we made the right decision."

Holly plans to move out of her parents' home. "My parents think that it's a good idea. They're not kicking me out. They just think it's a good idea. They think I'm going to resent them after, you know. It's my child. I should bring it up the way I want to. It's going to be different when I move out. Robert's been working a lot, so he really doesn't have enough time to see Neil, but he'll be able to see him every morning before he goes to work. But I'll be by myself all the time at the apartment, so I'll be going to my mom's.

"Sometimes I have doubts and say to Robert, 'Did we make the right decision?' and he'll say, "Look how beautiful he is. Of course we made the right decision.' "

We hear from Holly the challenge of being just eighteen, wanting her own birthday party and presents, and hoping her baby would not arrive to disrupt her personal celebration. We hear her wanting to please her parents and the baby's father. While taking the major responsibility for the baby, she wonders about the rightness of her decision. Teen mothers want to make the decision by themselves; yet they find, as Holly does, that the acting out of that decision is extremely difficult—they do sometimes have doubts.

ME AND SOMEBODY ELSE

Like older mothers, many teen mothers are fascinated by the experience of the baby in their bodies and the enjoyment of playing with the child once born. Carole says, "The really great time, the best feeling in the world, is the first time he smiles at you and it's a real smile. It's not a gas smile. It's just fantastic." Rachel, too, says "I figure that one of the most beautiful sounds there is, is listening to your child laugh." The connection to the child, the recognition that she is the mother, is what keeps the teen mother tied to her commitment to the child. Rachel talks of how important it is for her to be recognized as a mother.

Rachel O'Donnell. You and your daughter

Rachel went to be tested for pregnancy after missing her period. "I had a couple of dreams and in them I was pregnant. That's what made me think I was pregnant to begin with. I wasn't impressed. First of all, I didn't consent to it, so that really kind of shook me—that I was even pregnant to begin with." She has no contact with the father of the baby. "As far as he's concerned, I aborted it. My first thought was to abort it because of my age. But I didn't think I could go through with that. So then I decided I wouldn't do that. My mother was really encouraging me to abort it. She kept telling me it was a blob to try and make me feel better. By then I was about six weeks. And it's no longer a blob then. It's actually got all its little fingers and toes and things. And I considered giving it up for adoption. Then I found myself, I couldn't do that either. One of the reasons why I didn't go that way is because I don't think that I could look through all the books and find someone suitable. It was like, *it's your child*. I think we [meaning herself] made the right decision."

Although Rachel did not feel well throughout her pregnancy, it was a positive experience for her; she developed a strong relationship with her baby during her pregnancy. "He's got his own little personality. Sometimes he just rubs up against the side. And if you poke at him, he pokes back. Kind of like, 'give me room,' you know, 'don't cramp me . . . It's a really good feeling. Because you are going to bring something into the world. Then, of course, you can always laugh because the guys can't do it. Well, okay, yes, there's a lot of them that say that we've got to go through all that pain. I mean, they're missing out on a lot. It's a very warm feeling, I think."

Rachel's mother stayed with her through the entire labor. "I'd sleep in between contractions. Then I'd wake up. Mum would tell me to breathe, and she'd tell me that they were over. And I'd put my head down, and I'd go back to sleep. I'd wake up and I'd look over at her, her eyes were closed, and I tried to be really quiet, because I was hoping she'd be sleeping, because I felt so bad about keeping her there, and keeping her awake. She knew, and she'd start talking to me. They were cutting the cord and they were holding her up, and I could see a baby, but I saw legs and I saw nothing else except this little head itself. So mum told me it was a girl." [So despite Rachel's prediction, the baby was a girl.]

Three weeks after the birth, Rachel, her mother, and her daughter moved into their own place, primarily because Rachel's stepfather is an alcoholic. "It's working quite well," says Rachel, "I think it kind of comes naturally. I don't really see much of a change or problem with it. I mean, it's not like I was sacrificing a whole lot, because I wasn't one that would go out and party around anyway. To stay home with her hasn't really changed much. "I manage most of it. I insist on that. But I mean, then you've got times, like now when I'm sick, my mom does take care of her more and just little things like that. It's nice. My mom feeds her once in a while, and once in a while she changes her, but other than that, it's my responsibility. [But] when I'm sick, I tend to just do nothing. Mom takes care of Kate."

Rachel likes her new image of mother. "I was talking to someone on the phone. She said something about "you and your daughter,' and I figured that was one of the nicest things I've ever heard. It has a nice little ring, you know." Rachel is completing high school and, after doing a year of volunteer work at a youth emergency shelter, plans to attend college, where she will study to be a childcare worker. Rachel has Kate in daycare at her high school. "I usually feed her over lunch. Usually we play on the floor. It's nice though, because it gives you a little more quality time."

Rachel was not prepared for pregnancy. She did not consent to inter-course, and she says she was not impressed. She cried all the way home from the doctor's office. Yet, over her pregnancy she begins to get attached to her baby and finds that her life is better. She becomes more independent and gains great pleasure from her relationship to her daughter. She surprises herself.

Surprising Bodies

There is something curious, unexpected, even strange about being pregnant when pregnancy occurs completely at the wrong time. It seems that in today's society the teen years are definitely the wrong time for pregnancy. Pregnant teens' bodies are out of sync with sociocultural pressures and demands; they are out of sync with other teens' bodies. When a teen thinks, "it can never happen to me," perhaps it is because she is just getting comfortable with her own young, sexual body—the body that gets attention for its slimness and shapeliness. She cannot imagine her body any other way. The problem of not being able to button up her jeans comes as a surprise. Although many times a teen mother and her family keep the pregnancy a secret, eventually the secret becomes public. Her body eventually gives the secret away. The ability of her woman's body to be pregnant is not yet understood by the teenager, and therefore it comes as a surprise.

It is thought that teen mothers have an easier time than other mothers with the discomforts of pregnancy. Holly, however, has numerous problems. She says that her body is so small that the baby cannot move around without giving her severe backache. Celine also says that she has had the worst pregnancy—severe problems with morning sickness, anemia, nosebleeds, and has "gained fifty-six pounds so far." Teens talk of their experiences of their bodies as distinct from their experience of the baby. Their bodies are still their own.

Yet, having a baby in her body, as part of her body, is described as a pleasurable experience. Rachel takes great glee in talking to her baby inside. She describes her first sense of the baby as a "gurgle, like water boiling and you watch the bubbles come up, it kind of feels like that. When it kicks, and it's harder, your whole body moves from it. Other times he just rubs up against the side, and if I poke him, he pokes back. And if he decides he is hungry, he lets me know." She looks after her baby by eliminating bad habits, like coffee and chocolate. Ruth-Ann had a difficult time stopping drugs, especially cocaine, but says that now she does not "do drugs anymore." Others, like Holly, want to stop smoking, but find that they are unable to do so. Smoking was the most difficult habit to break, and they did not always succeed. They knew the implications and cut down on the number of cigarettes, but were not able to stop altogether. These teen mothers try to be responsible.

Birth itself brings more surprises—the time when labor starts, the length of labor, the degree of pain, and even making sure the right people are there.

For some teens labor and birth is an extremely painful, frightening experience. "The labor itself is like you've never experienced before—an atrocious pain," says Jesse. For others, labor is faster or easier than expected. Ruth-Ann says, "I don't think it was that hard. I didn't scream or anything." Labor and birth may have brought a deeper sense of confidence to some women. Jasmine knew she was in labor and knew she was ready to give birth, even though the nurses in the hospital would not believe her.

The one surprise that these teen mothers did not want was the possibility of something being wrong with the baby. Some were especially worried because of their behavior before they found out they were pregnant. "In the first trimester or whatever of your pregnancy, it's like the most important, because it's developing all its fingers and toes and everything. So I'm scared that there's going to be something wrong," says Jasmine. Her fear comes from the fact that before she found out she was pregnant she was "seriously drinking, I drank a lot, I think I was almost alcoholic, and I did drugs too—dope, acid. I'm scared. When I first got pregnant I just quit, just like that." Jasmine is critical of other girls she knows that do not seem to care, for they continue to take drugs and drink throughout their whole pregnancy. She says, "You're just ruining someone else's life. Doing it just because she wants to like keep all her friends and whatever—be cool, be popular."

Mother Material

Rachel developed her own vision of what it means to be *mother material*: a mother is not just a babysitter, but someone who teaches a child "right and wrong." Teaching a child is very different from having a cute baby to play with, or having a pet that may be around for a while. Teen mothers have to accomplish many things: finish school, establish a job or career, and, perhaps, find a partner. Teen mothers do not talk much about having a home of their own; they are usually still in their parents' home and on social assistance—at least for a while.

We have come to understand human growth and development in terms of the ability to become independent individuals valuing qualities of separation, differentiation, and autonomy (Carter and McGoldrick 1989). Erikson (1963), Piaget (1952), and Kohlberg (1981) built developmental theories that place positive value on these individualistic characteristics, largely from the point of view of male experience. For example, in Erik Erikson's (1963) eight stages of development, human connectedness is central to the first stage of life (trust versus mistrust), but does not appear again until the sixth stage (intimacy versus isolation). This emphasis on individuation throughout the life cycle has been challenged by the work of Carol Gilligan (1983), Jean Baker Miller (1986), Mary Belenky and her colleagues (1986), and others who point to women's development as being different from male development. Jean Baker Miller, a psychiatrist, describes woman's sense of self as organized around her ability to develop and maintain relationships, while Carol Gilligan suggests that a woman's moral development centers on characteristics of human attachment. The striving for relationship ("creating and sustaining relations of empathy and mutual intersubjectivity") may be considered as mature and essential as the striving for individual autonomy (Held 1990: 341).

If one evaluates the teen mother in terms of the development stages that have been identified by Erik Erikson (1963), she fails. She has jumped out of step. But if one evaluates her from the point of view of women's development, it may be that she is attempting to develop a healthy relational self (Miller and Stiver 1991). It may be that if viewed in terms of women's development, the teen mother's experience of having a child is more understandable and less abnormal. She is establishing a relationship with a child that helps her to succeed in learning more about herself and move toward further independence. Teen mothers are determined to mother their children well. They want to be "mother material," as Rachel wants to be. Rachel basks in the glow of the words "you and your daughter," words that place value on her connection to her baby, a relationship that she wants.

For Rachel, too, there is another connection that she values, a connection crucial for the teen mother. It is the relationship with her own mother—perhaps the best source of insight to the relational self that women have (Held 1990). The longing for relations with others, especially her own mother, is seen in the words of Jasmine, "We should be really close." Pregnancy for a teenager may not be seen as the usual developmental path, but it may be a path that is valuable for some young women.

At times teen mothers are torn between wanting to be mother material—being there to teach their baby right and wrong—and their desire to do things for themselves alone, things that other teens do without thinking. Ruth-Ann never leaves her baby, because she is breastfeeding, but she longs for the party life she used to have: "Sometimes I wish like I could go out and do things—be bad and stuff—stay out all night, like before, when I didn't have a care in my mind, wouldn't even care if my mom worried about me." Celine too struggles with her impulsiveness: "Sometimes, like if I see something I'll be impulsive and I'll just buy it." One thing that all teen mothers tend to agree on is that they are not having another baby for a long time. Teen mothers struggle to care for their child and still do things for themselves—a struggle all mothers face. To have time, energy, and support to take care both of your child and of yourself is a challenge for all mothers.

THREADBARE CONNECTIONS

Teen mothers are noticed when they walk in the mall or attend school. More often than not, it is not the kind of attention they want. Teen mothers are given a hard time by many people in the community—senior citizens, guys, school mates, and other women. Some people see teen mothers as a social problem or a drain on the public purse, and some even think they represent a decline in social morals. Not long ago, in my community a member of the government referred to single mothers as leeches who demand support money from the fathers of the children, and get pregnant in order to become supported by social welfare money. His comments created a public outcry, yet he is not alone in his attitudes. How do attitudes like these affect the experiences of teen mothers? How do attitudes like these affect the teen mother's ability to be the mother she wants to be?

In many ways, teen mothers are no different than other teens—worried about boys, about school, about relationships with parents, even about handling independence from parents. In other ways, they are different. It seems that many teen mothers are experiencing a particularly difficult time in their lives. While some teen mothers have troubled lives in troubled families, they all struggle with the pregnancy experience. It seems that for some of these teens the move toward independence took a wild turn toward outright rebellion—running away from school, away from parents, and/or away from home. For some teen mothers relationships (with boyfriends, parents, and school) are chaotic. There is turmoil in the home. There is turmoil in the school. There is alcohol and drug abuse, both their own and their parents'. Some describe poverty and breakups of relationships between parents. At fourteen Ruth-Ann had already run away from both her childhood home and a group home, because she "could not get along with her mother." Some teen mothers have bleak stories, indeed. They are frustrated with most relationships in their lives and feel, as Celine does, that no one gives them a break.

Celine Merrill. Nobody wants to give me a break!

Celine did not really expect that she would be able to get pregnant. But by age fifteen she had already had a miscarriage. While not actually planned, Celine thinks a pregnancy would "fill the gap." "I think I wanted to undo what I did wrong because of my first pregnancy. If I had known I was pregnant [the first time], I would not have done half the things that I was doing. I felt really guilty."

Celine also thinks her boyfriend, William, wants a baby. He thinks a baby would help him gain respect from his parents, make them "treat him like a human being." William is twenty-three. Celine thinks "it is time." She did think about adoption, weighing the pros and cons, but decided that "it's not like I'm really going to be a single parent, because William's going to be there with me. He's always telling me he loves me lots." Celine is comfortable with having a baby at sixteen. "I know it's a natural occurrence and, like, the majority of women do get pregnant. It's just I'm doing it at an earlier age. We still have the same health risks. And, like, every pregnancy is different, but we still go through the same things. Like, our stomachs get bigger and then we have a baby. But I wouldn't mind being a couple of years older, because then things would come easier to me. Like, Social Services would help me automatically and stuff like that. One thing that really bothers me is the way people look at you. They look at you like you're a sideshow freak. I was walking in the mall with my friend, and she was pregnant as well. We got called "sluts" from this old man. You know, it's ignorance on their part, because fifty years ago sixteen-year-old girls were getting pregnant."

Celine has little contact with her mother. She ran away from home. "The last night that I spent in the house with my mother," she says, "this woman [her mother], who weighs three hundred pounds, sat on me for an hour and a half. I didn't want to listen to her insulting me. So she sat on me so she could insult me and I'd have to listen." Celine says she has been abused by her mother throughout her life, and says that she does not" want my child to go through the same abuse that I did." Her real father died drinking and driving. Her mother married his best friend, Jack, who was like a father to Celine. "He was so bright, he read books all the time, and he could have been someone. But because of drugs and alcohol he's a nobody. He's a bum on the streets. And I don't want, I don't want, I don't want my life to be like that. And I don't want my life, my child, to be like that. It's just not for me."

Celine calls William "her knight in shining armor," who got her out of her mother's place by inviting her to live at his parents' home. Celine lived there for about four months, until William's mother decided that she could no longer support her. She lived in many different places, ending up for most of her pregnancy in a residence for young pregnant women. Celine often feels badly treated and fights over rules and curfews. "They treat me like garbage," she says. She is asked to leave the residence just three days after giving birth to Jenny. "It just seems like nobody wants to give me a break. So I was a sixteen-year-old girl with a three-day old baby, and I had nowhere to go." She was initially placed in a foster home, but was then granted independent status and moved into an apartment of her own.

Before the baby's birth, Celine didn't know what it was going to be like to be a mother, but was confident in her ability to care for her baby. "I'm capable of being a mother just as well as a thirty-year-old is. In actuality, I'm probably more responsible than a lot of adults out there. I babysat ever since I was about eleven years old. Like, I get along with kids great, you know. I'm able to discipline kids without yelling at them, or hitting them, or anything like that. I don't think that it's going to be as hard as everybody says it is. I think I am mature enough, and that I'm responsible enough that I can take care of my child."

After Jenny is born, Celine finds her life has changed somewhat, but "not so dramatically that I've noticed it. You know, it's just, it's almost natural for me. It didn't seem really any different. It was just someone else there. Breastfeeding's a breeze, 'cause all you do is stick her there and you go back to sleep." She is aware of the responsibilities of caring for and safeguarding Jenny. She has already faced the challenges of colic, immunizations, and financial responsibilities. "She scared me last night. Holy smokes! I almost died of a heart attack. I was going to lay her down to feed her. All of a sudden she had this really weird look on her face and she wasn't breathing, so I picked her up and I started smacking her on the back. And, oh, a big chunk of sour milk came out." Celine does not regret her decision. "I kind of wonder what my life would be now if I didn't have her. I can't imagine what I would miss. It just scares me to think of what I would have missed if I had an abortion."

Four months after Jenny's birth, William continues to live with his parents for financial reasons. He provides some financial and social support to Jenny and Celine. Celine, however, feels that in some ways she supports William and that he is not always as helpful as she wishes. "He uses breastfeeding as an excuse not to hold her and stuff like that. Around his family, he's the model father, you know, but around here he doesn't do much." Many of William's close relatives still do not know about Jenny, nor has Celine informed her own mother.

Celine started correspondence courses right after Jenny's birth. She intends to finish high school and go on to university. She has applied for daycare at school and expects to get it because breastfeeding women get priority. She wants to become a pediatrician.

It is clear that Celine has had a difficult time establishing a place for herself—running away from home, living in many different foster-type situations, staying in a home for pregnant teens, eventually achieving independent status and living with her tiny baby in an apartment by herself. It is remarkable that teen mothers like Celine have the ability and tenacity to keep searching for the support they need. They are not lazy. Celine at fifteen looks after herself. In many ways, she, especially, seems very much alone in getting what she needs to care for herself and her baby.

Although the teen mothers frequently suggest that being a mother at sixteen is no different than being a mother at thirty, their talk shows the reality of their age. Celine wants to go back to a regular high school for grade twelve because she wants a graduation. The school for teen mothers, with its particular supports such as individualized programming and childcare facilities, does not have the kind of graduation activities that Celine imagines for herself. Holly stays home Saturday nights and wishes she could be like her friends, partying and having fun. Robert, her baby's father, thinks Holly is boring, and she begins to think so as well. Ruth-Ann wants to go out and have fun. There are no dances at the school she attends, and she wishes there were. She says, "Even if I have a baby, I could go to dances." These mothers, like all other mothers, want to be who they uniquely are outside of the role of mother.

The teen mothers remark as well that having a baby at a young age now is no different than it was fifty years ago. But, of course, it is different. In earlier days, the community was supportive, women were married at sixteen, and pregnancy was expected of them. Now, the lack of community support is evident. Indeed, these teen mothers experience criticism from every direction—the negative and hostile looks, the whispers, the name-calling, the feeling of being a "sideshow freak," and being told what to do. Rachel talks of the looks, "those" looks, looking down at you because you shouldn't be that way, kind of thing." Many older pregnant women in our society experience the opposite—the congratulations, the smiles, and the protection. The physical experience of older and younger mothers may be similar, yet the reality of being a teen mother is much more difficult, with less support by the community. Not only does she get less social support, she often gets outright criticism.

We often talk of the need for a social safety net to assist people through difficult circumstances in their lives—including young women becoming mothers. Much of the time the social safety net is conceived of as the financial support that is necessary to keep people fed and sheltered. But a social safety net needs more than just money. The current social safety net for teen mothers is threadbare and tattered when it does not include the kind words and encouraging nods that reward the positive mothering actions of these mothers. Celine talks of the delight she experienced in this regard. One evening, when the baby was very young, Celine and William went to a movie with their baby. The baby was quiet the whole time. The woman who sat in front of them said to Celine after the movie, "Oh what a sweet baby. She's just so quiet. I can't believe it. I never heard a baby like that before. You're a model to every mother." Celine glows as she tells me. She says, "I loved it. I was walking on air for about a day." The social safety net surrounding this young mother supported her in ways that are less tangible but as important as the provision of money.

School Days

School is important to teen mothers: it is their job. The school the teen mothers I spoke to attended was created just for them. It has programs arranged to accommodate the childcare needs of these mothers, with flexible schedules, daycare support, counseling, and other educational sessions. Many teen mothers find it difficult to continue at regular high schools, as other teens do not accept their pregnancy and there is no support for the care of their babies. The notion of pregnancy and babies is outside of the expectations or even imaginations of some schoolmates in regular schools. Jasmine says of her grade nine class at school, "I don't think people think about sex at my school."

School is important. Not one of the teen mothers that I spoke to dropped out of school once she was pregnant. In fact, once pregnant they all returned to school, and some of them had aspirations to go to college or university. Ruth-Ann talks of her need for direction and deadlines. She says she needs more push: "I'm not pushed enough. Like, they don't push you enough. It's whenever you're done, hand it in. I can't. I just don't do it. You know, what's the use of doing it if you're not going to be pushed towards anything? That's the way I see it." For Ruth-Ann, the flexible independent study style does not work as well as she would like, so she plans to go back to a regular high school for grade ten.

The school for teen mothers is a place of support. It is a nonjudgmental environment where teen mothers can finish high school, learn parenting and general life skills, and have their children well cared for in daycare. Schools like this one provide an excellent foundation for teen mothers before and after the birth of their children. In a northern community, where the old way of having the extended family care for a teen mother's child has broken down, a teen parent program offers an encouraging environment that will help break the cycle of poverty and despair of these mothers and their babies (Hayden 1995).

The Father of the Baby

Although the babies' fathers are sometimes in the background or periphery of the teen mothers' picture, they are rarely solidly in the frame. The fathers mentioned by the women in this study are not teens themselves, but tend to be several years older than the mothers. The relationships between these parents are unsettled. Often the teen mothers feel that the baby's father does not care either about the baby or about them. Statements like "he's not interested," "has other babies behind my back," or "threatens to take the baby" show the nature of many of the relationships. Other fathers, like William O'Brien, who feels he will get more respect from his own parents as a parent himself, and Robert Alder, who does not want his baby to grow up in a single-parent family, are committed to their babies and the mothers. In this study group, however, the parents did not live together as a family.

Jasmine says, "The father—we broke up before I found out I was pregnant, a month before. He was still calling me and stuff. He is a threat. He knows I'm pregnant and stuff, but he doesn't want to pay any money for child support. He doesn't care. He keeps on saying stupid things like 'I'm going to steal the baby. I'm going to get custody of it,' but I know he never would." Rachel says of the father of her baby, 'I don't want him in my life, and I don't want to deal with a child that's upset with broken promises, because he'd be one of these fathers that would make plans and break them." None of the teen mothers with whom I spoke had a happy, secure, stable partnership. Rachel was raped and the baby's father thought she had an abortion. Although Holly had broken up with Robert, they are now attempting to work out a good relationship. The father of Jasmine's baby still threatens to take her. William, the father of Celine's baby, at twenty-three lives in his parents' home, has two jobs, is paying off debts and buying a new car. While he visits often and takes some part in the care of the child, the primary responsibility for the care and support of the child is Celine's. A year after my last interview with Celine, she informed me that her relationship with William was shaky. Before her son's birth, Ruth-Ann does not know if the father is white or black, and says, "Can't expect him to stick around or anything, can't expect that from anybody." After the birth (when she knows who the father is), Ruth-Ann wishes she had not told him about the baby. She wrote a letter to him in jail and told him that the baby was born. "But," she says, "that was a stupid thing to do. I thought maybe, like, he'd be nice and stuff. Maybe he would like to see him. But then he started saying that he's going to get custody of Wylie. That frightened me." While the fathers' experience is not pursued in this research, from the point of view of the teen mothers, relationships with the babies' fathers are often precarious and troubled. Even if the fathers are in the picture, the teen mothers shoulder the primary responsibility for the care of the child.

Needing a Mother

"If I was to live alone I don't think I would be able to handle it. I'd get very upset. I'd be scared to live alone—the way I'd react sometimes," says Ruth-Ann, who lives in a housing unit with her mother. While Ruth-Ann does most of the childcare, her mother does most of the other household duties, such as cooking, cleaning, and laundry. The relationship of the teen mothers with their own mothers is very important: it is central to their lives. Teen mothers benefit from their mothers' support and guidance. They want it and value it. They want their mothers' advice about how to look after their babies; they do not want them to take over the care, but to give ideas and backup. They need their mothers to help them in their mothering. "I need my mom because, you know, I can't raise a newborn baby by myself, I don't know the first thing about it. She does," says Jasmine.

Yet support for pregnancy, birth, and parenting is not the only thing that the teen wants from her mother. Teen years are a time of personal change, of distancing from the influence of her mother, of testing independence, and of rebellion and questioning. Yet teens need their mothers to stay close. Although Celine left home before her pregnancy, she seems to be searching for a mother, finding mothers at her boyfriend's and a girlfriend's home, at a foster home, and at a temporary group home. None of these "mothers" is quite right, or perhaps none is willing or able to be the mother that Celine seeks. The teen mother needs her mother for herself. She needs caring and loving when she is sick, not only to help with the baby. She needs company, someone to talk to, to fill empty hours. She needs guidance for growing up. Jasmine begs her mother to be a mother to her, wishing that she would stay home, that she would not drink, and even that she would go to social services with her. She says, "I still need my mom there. I'm still young too. I'm still her baby, so I still need help from her and she still has to do things for me, like for my cold and take care of me." These teen mothers say they grew up overnight, but in some ways they do not grow up fast enough. They still need their mothers, perhaps more than ever.

The teen mother needs someone to challenge her, someone to take on the role of mother, to ground her, to situate her experience of being a teenager. She needs a role model to test, someone to compare herself with, to measure against. Am I like my mother? Do I want to be like my mother? The frustrations that Holly experiences in living at home and following curfews are part of the teenage experience, ways of growing up through her relationship with her mother. "They're so overprotective now," says Holly. "I mean, I can't even go out at night. They like to know exactly where I am. I mean, I'm eighteen years old, and I went out to the bar about four months before I even got pregnant. I didn't come home half the time, and they didn't care."

Rachel and her mother work together to make this new life good for them. Once Rachel decided to keep her baby, her mother supported her through all the hard as well as the enjoyable parts of pregnancy, birth, and caring for the baby. Rachel says she has the best mother. Her mother joined her in exercises, prenatal classes, and other preparations for the new baby. Rachel says, "I think I'm about the only one that has a mother quite like mine. She's an angel. I don't know what I'd do without her. You should see her. She plays with my cats and she talks to them weird. I keep telling her she needs a grandchild. Parents, you know, you get them around kids and instant mush."

Rachel's mother took part in all our conversations, and says that this pregnancy has made a difference in Rachel's life. She says of Rachel, "She has grown a lot. Whether she has realized that or not. She's always been independent and what not, but it's given her another drive and another reason to definitely go out and say, 'well, this is what I have to do in the future, because I not only have me, but I have someone else to take care of too.' It's made a difference." Here we see another side of the growth to independence. Through her experience of the relationship with her baby, Rachel is moved to follow her own goals. In the move to independence through relationship, these young mothers need their own mothers, or someone else, to assist them. Teen mothers need the care and support that all teens need.

Being a mother, yet needing a mother, is the challenge. Wanting and needing help, yet needing to assert her role as the mother to her baby, has potential for confusion and conflict in a mother's relationship with her own mother. Holly's mother encourages her to move out so that she can have the opportunity to raise Neil in her own way. Her parents do not want Holly to resent them for wanting to raise the child their way. Holly thinks finding her own place is a good idea, but worries about being alone all day and about not having her mother to take Neil for even a few minutes each day. She says, "Now, when my mom comes home, she basically looks after Neil for half an hour because she hasn't seen him all day. That gives me half an hour just to do whatever I want." Jasmine struggles against her mother's referring to *our* baby and her gentle threats to keep Jade if Jasmine wants to move away. Yet, Jasmine acknowledges that she needs her mother, especially when she is sick. Celine is not able to resolve her difficult relationship with her mother during pregnancy, and consequently does not inform her about Jenny's birth.

Mothers and daughters have an important relationship, which is often highlighted during a daughter's pregnancy and when a baby comes into her life. Teen mothers are not only learning ways to separate from their mothers in order to find their own unique selves, but also facing a situation where they need their mothers to be with them in the same ways that any teenager does. Teen mothers need a wise mother—a wise grandmother—who will know when to step in to assist, and when to step away to support her daughter to find her own original way.

GOOD MOTHERS

This morning I fed him at five and then we slept for a while. I know I'm not supposed to do this, but usually if he eats at five and I want to go back to sleep, I'll just put him in my arm and go to sleep with him there because he sleeps so good with me. He'll just go to sleep because he is so relaxed and warm with his mommy. (Carole Benson)

The teen mothers in this study are well aware of the enormity of their responsibility in deciding to keep the baby, but it is only after the birth that the responsibility becomes real to them. Caring for her child requires sacrifices and lifestyle changes for every mother. For teen mothers, it may mean giving up drinking, partying, or even just going out shopping whenever they want. It means being different than other teens. For these teen mothers, it means going to a school particularly for them and spending their lunchtime with their babies in the school daycare. It means being up at night to feed and soothe a crying baby. It means doing homework while someone else, usually their own parents, look after the baby—but still feeling responsible if the baby cries. It means trusting yourself, like Carole does, in spite of what experts might tell you, in having the baby sleep with you.

All the teen mothers in this study got pregnant by mistake or as an accident—by thinking pregnancy could never happen to them (it hadn't happened before!), by forgetting to take the birth control pills, by being raped, or by not having condoms available. A couple of the teens thought they would probably never be able to become pregnant due to some childhood accident or illness. Whatever the reason, everyone is surprised. Like Sally Corbett, a placing mother, these teen mothers say, "I was shocked." Perhaps, one might think, they should not be so surprised. They should know better. Some of these young women talk of their behavior—being wild, having unprotected sex, drinking excessively, using drugs, never coming home, partying, not caring about anything, school, parents, and so on. To be sexually active from twelve or thirteen is common. Many of these teens think that their parents did not care—perhaps they think nobody cares.

To think of their pregnancy as a mistake is different than thinking that these teen mothers are bad. Talking with these young pregnant women, so lovely, so honest, yes, so giggly, perhaps naive and unrealistic about what it takes to be a mother (as many mothers are), made me think about their abilities and their needs. Seeing them bring their babies to our meetings with all the necessary supports—car seats, blankets, bottles, diaper bags, and so on—showed me their abilities and responsibilities. Having the baby changes the behavior of many teen mothers, at least during pregnancy and early mothering. Rachel says, "My driving's improved. It is not just me, it's me and my baby. Not just me I'm looking out for anymore." In some ways, growing up with their babies may have saved their lives. Jasmine says, "I changed totally. I just changed totally. If I hadn't gotten pregnant, who knows where I would've been now. Not home, that's for sure."

Jasmine Jonson. I was so bad

Jasmine was fifteen, in grade nine at school, when she found out that she was pregnant. Although she had been sexually active since thirteen, and involved with her boyfriend for seven months, she was not using birth control measures. She was shocked. "I didn't think it could happen to me." Jasmine's first plan is to have an abortion. Her mother thinks Jasmine should just forget about her pregnancy, so that "things will just get back to normal." But, especially after the ultrasound, Jasmine decides to keep the baby—which is what she really wanted all along: "If I did that [abort the baby], I'll always be wondering what the kid looked like and what it would be like. Now I don't think I'd ever consider having an abortion."

Jasmine's labor is fast. She knows her baby is about to be born even though the nurses do not believe her. Her mother, father, aunt, and some friends accompany her to the hospital. "They were outside and they were watching through this window, and then they just came in when they saw the head coming out. She just came out really fast." Jasmine and her mother argue over naming the baby. "She wants me to name the baby a name she likes and I don't like. Like, it's my choice, it's my child." She names her daughter Jade.

Jasmine has minimal contact with her baby's father during pregnancy or after the birth. He is seven years older, nonsupportive, threatens to take the child, and has a criminal record, Jasmine says. She wishes he would just disappear. "He's a total idiot, total."

Jasmine, the oldest of three girls, lives at home. Sometimes she gives up her bed when her aunt comes to stay. Now she says she doesn't do drugs at all, while before the pregnancy she says she was seriously drinking, and doing dope and acid. Now she sometimes has a drink, because she says she comes from a family of drinkers: "my dad's a drinker, my mom's a drinker, all my aunts and uncles are drinkers." Her father, "not the kind of person to tell his feelings, is responsible," thinks Jasmine, "he only drinks on the weekends." But she longs for a closer relationship with her mother. During pregnancy, Jasmine says, "We should be really close. My mother goes out all of the time. I have no one to talk to. I just stay at home and do nothing. She always goes out. I just want her company once in a while, you know. She's always going out. She's always getting totally drunk." Jasmine must do everything on her own. "What happens," questions Jasmine, "if I go into labor and she's at the bar or something? I've tried to phone her there and page her, but they don't let you." Jasmine worries that her ten-year-old twin sisters will turn out just like her—bad. And while she wants her mother to be with her more, she also worries that she will try to control or possess her baby. She says, "It's just that she's already saying it's *our* baby or *my* baby. It's not. I'm the one that's having it."

Jasmine felt out of place in her old school, and changed to a high school for young pregnant women and single mothers. She feels the weight of the responsibility of being pregnant, of being a mother. She sees older women staring at her and thinking, "poor her, look at her. It's so hard. But really I don't think it's much different for any woman. It's still the same responsibility coming on. You miss going out a lot, but she's still a good thing. I'd rather have her than have any social life for sure." Jasmine is completely responsible for Jade's care. "You get to grow up with her. I would never give her away. Ever." While Jasmine hopes to find a way to live independently from her family, she knows that she can't right now. "But," she says, "I won't stay with them that long. My mom's just too . . . she just tells me what to do. It gets on my nerves. I know I'm going to be leaving one of these days.

"I used to be pretty bad. I drank and everything. I was so bad. I didn't think, nobody thought, I would change ever. And then as soon as I found out I was pregnant, I stopped. I started going to school again and then, I don't know, I just changed totally. I've learned a lot about school and about men and I don't know, how much cheaters they can be. I'm planning to stay away from men for a long time. I'm going to be a single parent, have safe sex, not going to run around like that ever again. I will go to school until I get to university and take English Literature. That is my plan."

She finished grade nine with honors.

Giving life to a child saved her life, thinks Jasmine. She wonders where she would be without Jade. When I first met Jasmine, she seemed like a lost little girl. Later, after her baby was born, she seemed much stronger and more sure of herself. She has plans for her life. She says she changed so totally that even she seems surprised. Is her change just a behavioral change, a practical and social change, or is it something deeper? Is it a moral change, one that comes with her turning toward her child and brings her power through her connection to her baby girl? Rachel says, "It is not just me I'm looking out for anymore." Lee SmithBattle speaks about Tammy, another teen mother; "The world of mothering works a moral change in Tammy's life, giving birth to a relational self, a self born out of emerging skills, meaning, and habits of caring for and responsiveness to a specific child" (1994: 150). Teen mothers move to change their behavior because of their connection to their child, a relationship that causes them to think about what they should do and how they should behave.

Strengths

From seeking confirmation of the pregnancy to telling family and friends, changing schools, facing changes in her body, facing labor, and then raising her child, the teen mother has to call upon her strengths over and over. She is challenged. Sometimes she is supported by others—family, friends, boyfriends, schools—and sometimes she is questioned by family, the social welfare system, and professionals. Sometimes she has to do things alone and sometimes she has considerable support. Celine at a very young age was able to negotiate her way around the welfare system, finally finding a place to live with her daughter. Imagine the strength that she needed to stay with her dream of mothering Jenny when she found herself without a place to live in when her baby was only three days old. Perhaps there is a temptation to give up, to leave Jenny, to place her for adoption—which we know can also be a strength. It is not an option Celine wants to take. Her strength may be a kind of growing up, a stretching toward maturity or a way of finding maturity.

For the teen mother, strength may come from her pregnancy or from events in her life before the pregnancy. Rachel and her mother were already facing turmoil in their lives, making a decision about moving away from the stepfather, who was an alcoholic. These young women needed to find strength to make hard decisions, to make major changes in their lives, and to face unpleasant realities that were already a part of their lives. They found the strength to focus on what needs to be done and getting it done, "focus on the future, and one step at a time," as Celine says. These young women realized that in order to hold on to their visions, to create a life that fit those visions, it was sometimes necessary to stand up to others, like their parents or the baby's father. Holly's father at first demanded that she abort her child. Holly did not comply and stayed with her decision, which her parents later supported. It was sometimes necessary to adjust, revise plans, and make different arrangements. During pregnancy most of these teen mothers had ideas of how much school they could be attending after the baby was born, but needed to make adjustments to those plans once the baby was born—changing expectations of completion dates and rearranging course loads. Yet, all continued working at their schoolwork in some way. The high school diploma and the possibility of university or college stayed part of the vision.

Loving Children and Mothers

Mothers need to be heard, cared for, and understood, says Jane Swigart (1991), and their need is as important as that of the child. "Most children cannot be helped if mothers are not helped and supported" (Swigart 1991: 2). Becoming and being a mother—a good mother—is difficult and requires hard work and commitment. Being a good mother means protecting, providing for, and teaching the baby. For the teen mother it means keeping her baby safe—making a home, buying a crib, knowing what to do if her baby is choking, finding the right babysitters, creating the right family, often without the support of her baby's father. Being a mother is more than being just a babysitter. It means teaching the child right and wrong. The reality of taking care of a child, loving a child, during all those days and all those nights, during all those hours and all those minutes, needs to be acknowledged. However much teen mothers, indeed all mothers, want to be perfect mothers, we need to acknowledge that "there are no perfect mothers on this earth" (Swigart 1991: 7). There are no perfect children. There are no perfect homes. In fact, searching for perfection leads us in the wrong direction. Rachel gives a hint of the myth of the perfect mother as she thinks of searching through the files of adoptive parents for the perfect mother for her child. She knows she will not be able to find anyone suitable, "because you could [always] find anything wrong with them. Just any little, little, itty picky something will be wrong with everybody. It would be hard to find the right parent for your child." She knows that if she looked for the perfect mother she would never find one; so, she seems to think, she might as well keep her baby to raise herself. She knows she will not be the perfect mother either, yet she wants to be a good one. But even the notion that there is a *good* mother, that all-giving nurturing mother, and a *bad* mother, that self-absorbed, inadequate, blameworthy mother (Swigart 1991), needs to be critically examined. Rather than focusing on good or bad, perfect or imperfect, one should listen to and compassionately understand the *real* mother, a mother with both her bright and her dark side.

In writing their story, in speaking their truth, teen mothers have two plots—the growth and development of their babies and the growth and development of themselves. Teen mothers are growing up with their babies. As the teen mother reflects, criticizes, searches to find the mother within her, she looks for guidance from her own mother, her friends, her family, and the other people around her. She needs and wants to be seen as the child's growing, learning, and loving mother. She feels the weight of the opinions, the stares of others. Whispers of "slut" or "too young" speak loudly to her, always questioning her ability and expecting her to fail. People generally expect mothers to be good mothers; yet, when it comes to teen mothers, it almost seems as if people are waiting for them not to be good enough. The teen mother is the learning mother, the changing mother, the mother who gains support by strong, loving whispers of approval—"Oh what a sweet baby. You're a model to every mother!"

Teen mothers realize that the connection they have with their child cannot be easily broken. We learn from Jasmine what this connection to her child does for her. As she begins to mother her baby, Jade, she worries about her own sisters. She worries that they will end up the same way as she did. She sees that they need a mother to keep them safe. All mothers need to have a supportive environment "to counter a society that is in many respects inimical to the well-being of both children and their care-givers" (Swigart 1991: 3). Such an environment, like a strongly textured blanket, would wrap around mothers and their children to provide space, support, warmth, and love for them. Children, and society, need mothers—not perfect mothers, because there are none, but *real* mothers, as true to themselves and their children as they can be.

In the final chapter I will explore how the experience of mothering can inform our understanding of our moral commitments to each other. I postulate that through the experience of pregnancy, childbirth, and nurturing we are morally moved to respond to the children in our lives. This response, which is profoundly experienced by mothers, is available to all who come to have a child on their mind. The experience of pregnancy, both for the child and the mother, is the place where human relationship begins.

NOTE

I wish to acknowledge the assistance of Susan James, Midwife and PhD Candidate, Faculty of Nursing, University of Alberta, in the writing of this chapter.

5

The Way of the Mother

The nature of the mother is shown in the words of the women who become mothers. Each mother is distinctive and comes to mothering in a unique and individual way; yet mothers speak in voices that resonate with other mothers. Many times in mothering the commitment to the child occurs easily, is done willingly and lovingly. It is a commitment, a devotion that often catches the woman unawares, before she has a chance to be rational about it. She is caught by the child in her body, in her heart, and in her mind. Other times, the commitment does not come so easily, especially when troubling factors enter the picture—lack of support from partners, family, or community; too many things to do; inadequate finances to provide for the child; or insufficient life experience to know how best to care for a child. However and whenever the commitment of a mother to her child occurs, it needs to be supported. Commitment to children needs to be fostered by the community where the mother lives.

In this chapter I explore what can be learned from the experience of the commitment that mothers have for their children. I propose that *the way of the mother* has to do not only with relations between women and children, but also with the social fabric of society, which affects relations between men and children, friends and neighbors, acquaintances and strangers. What I mean is that the relation between mother and child, a relation necessary for the health and growth of children, is the natural ground of the impulse toward a morality of responsibility, toward thinking of the other person as well as oneself—the move from *me, me, me* to *us*. When I use the word "impulse," I think of an impetus or trigger that starts something moving that is already in place. The instinct (energy or knowledge), the innate ability to be attentive and loving to others as well as ourselves, is already there. In taking the moral pulse of our society, it may be well to attend to the way we treat children and the mothers (whether they are birth mothers, adopting, or nurturing) who care for children on a day-to-day basis. The questions that frame this chapter are these: What is the knowledge that mothers learn, through their experience of turning toward the child, that can be learned by all of us? What can *the way of the mother* teach us? What is the teaching?

First, I explore the claim of the child as a moral claim. I suggest that the experience of women during pregnancy, birth, and nurturance demonstrates how the woman turns toward the child, and how, in this turning to the child (as Other), she comes to a renewed sense of herself (the Self). In this moral turn the woman asks the questions, "Who am I?" and "What should I do now?" Using reproductive choices as an example, I propose that moral questions and our responses to them stem from a relational root—the commitment that we have toward each other. Within the concept of freedom and choice we face the freedom of morality—to choose one behavior over another. The freedom to choose children is something that we all share. The choice of mothering (indeed, parenting) needs a societal commitment and an environment where children are valued. The chapter will conclude with a discussion of the power of the story (narrative) as a way to uncover, recover, and reimagine the story of the mother and how her story affects us all. I suggest that the stories of mothering are sources of moral knowledge. To begin this exploration, I turn again to the narratives of the women with whom I learned.

THE CLAIM OF THE CHILD

I guess it is just that they are helpless and you really feel that you have to care for them. And also when Lisa came out, she opened her eyes and had a very good long look at both Jim and I—very intelligently—almost as if she recognized us by our voices or something. It's just so overwhelming. You can't turn her down. (Jane Gibson)

Research on mothers and mothering has largely focused on maternal roles, psychological adaptations, developmental tasks, female identity formation, and, most extensively, issues of bonding and attachment. The goal of such research is to define mothering, to pin it down, so to speak, and therefore to be able to evaluate how well women measure up: "Has the mother accepted her maternal role?" "Has she adapted?" "Has she bonded with her child?" "Is she a good mother?" This kind of research moves professionals to question themselves and their services: "How can we help her accept her maternal role?" "Will having the newborn stay with the mother for one hour or two be important?" On one level, such questions are appropriate and valuable, aimed at supporting women to become better mothers. On another level, they are judgmental and evaluative of mothers, especially those who do not fit into well-defined parameters.

Research that attempts to understand women's experience of becoming mother as seen from their point of view has a different focus. This focus has been called the *science of wisdom*, as it attempts to reveal knowledge to show us how to live rather than to pin knowledge down in order to control life (Capra and Steindl-Rast 1991). Research that explores women's narratives about their own experience of becoming mother does not attempt to explain actions, to divide these actions into categories, to identify deficits and failures, to label experiences as tasks, roles, or adaptations, or to evaluate mothers as good or bad, or their activities as right or wrong. Rather, this research searches for an understanding of what a woman goes through as she becomes a mother. The experience of coming to have *a child on her mind* is relational at its root, and being relational it has to do with morality. As with any question of morality, this experience involves a self-question, "How should I act now?" rather than a statement, "This is how you should act now!" We have seen this relational commitment change Jasmine Jonson's behavior when she says, "And then as soon as I found out I was pregnant, I stopped. I started going to school again and then, I don't know, I just changed totally." Jasmine at fifteen is a teacher. Are we ready to hear her commitment to her child and to support her? Are we ready to learn from her?

The central mothering themes identified in this research are the experiences of: (1) deciding to become a mother and how that will be lived; (2) the lifelong presence (and absence) of the child (fetus, infant, etc.); (3) the intense feelings of love, pain, and fear associated with birth, placement, adoption, and the care of the child; and (4) the responsibility of having a child in one's life for a long time. These themes turn our attention to the lived reality of mothering, of how to live with and for the child and still maintain one's own life. But this focus on who mothers are and what experiences they have cannot be divorced from the reality of living, as a mother, in a cultural and social world. So while it may appear that only mothers—women who bring children into their lives—are faced with the question "How should I live now?" this is a question we all share. Individually and communally, we must face the same relational question of how we turn toward the child and toward one another. But when we ask the moral question of what we should be doing when faced with the children in our lives, it is not to point with shame or blame. Rather, it is to point to possibilities and to the meaning of human life. What does being (or having) a mother mean to my life? What does having (or being) a child mean to my life?

We are all born of a mother. We are all born into the physical (natural, biological) and social (cultural) world of relational commitments. "We cannot escape from our relational nature" and to think we can "is one of the great illusions of modernity" (Schultz and Carnevale 1992: 201). Being born of a woman is the primordial experience of relationship. It is *the* relationship on which all other relationships are built. That is why the mothering relation is so important to consider, to understand, and to value. In the mothering relation the biological and the cultural become mixed up. It is here that the mind and the body are one. A baby is born in and through the woman's body, but the baby is born in and through her culture as well. If the birth mother cannot care for the child, someone else—another mother, another person—can and must. The child is a child of us all. We are all responsible.

What about the woman's body as home? The possibility of such a notion is evident in the unreflective words of a twelve-year-old boy as he sits on his mother's lap, "You know, this is my home." He and his mother are playing around with how he used to be held in her lap, laughingly trying the different positions his preadolescent body can no longer comfortably fit—a body around which his mother can scarcely see. This boy is not talking about the *home* of the kitchen where they are playing. Rather, Sem is speaking of his *first* home, the body of his mother. The body of mother, as first home, as the first grounding and experience of love and connection originates a love not sentimental or romantic, but a love so elaborate, complex, and dependable that it supports the fetus to grow and become a child. With this profound love, there is a cultural responsibility to support it, to encourage mothers in it, to value it, and to foster its unfolding. The mother and child relation is important in itself, that is, for the individual mother and child, and yet it is important for us all.

What kind of a world is a good home for a child? The National Film Board production of *Expectations* by Suzanne Gervais (1993) shows a woman, nine months pregnant, happily awaiting the birth of her child. As the short video unfolds, her happiness changes to fear. We feel this fear as a ripe pear slips from her grasp landing by sharp-pointed, aggressively positioned scissors. This ominous image triggers in the woman a recognition of the danger that the world holds for her unborn child. In the film the pregnant woman expresses and transforms her anxiety by using her camera to capture the images of the life around her—images filled with shadows, barbed-wire fences, war, and bombs. These are anxieties that mothers face, anxieties we all face. The images are real. As women become mothers, they become aware of the world as home for the child. They become concerned about the world in a different way than before—as Rachel O'Donnell, a seventeen-year-old mother, says, "It is no longer just me I have to think about."

Is our world a good place for children? Does the experience of the mother, like Gervais's images in the mind of the pregnant woman, remind us to attend to the world as a place for children? In writing about the mothers of

Jerusalem, the poet Di Brandt writes about mothers, no matter where, in a way they can understand.

> every Friday the women gather in Jerusalem
> wearing black, holding roses instead of guns, to
> protest their sons & brothers becoming killers, their
> husbands coming home at night, tight lipped, tossing
> in bed, feverish, moaning, their aging fathers mean
> & hard with anger, shouting, arguing with everyone,
> with God, the women silent against them, wearing
> black, holding roses, heartsick, against the tide of
> blood flowing through Israel, is this the kind of
> homeland we wanted, is the kind of sons &
> daughters we wanted, hard, embittered, scarred? (1995: 24)

The relational commitment learned through mothering—the being with and for the Other and the being with and for the self—needs to be cherished. So while the wisdom learned by mothering is primarily for the mother and child (a particular mother and child), it is also for all of us—creating the possibility of a full life, a morally lived life—and thus for life itself. Valuing the way of the mother could save the homeland, could save the world as our homeland. Becoming and being a mother occurs in the world and is mediated by the context in which the mother lives. Being a mother is biological and cultural at the same time; yet it is not biologically determined, for it can be culturally changed (Nelson 1995). The aim of this chapter is to remind us all that such a context, a world where the mothering relation can flourish, needs to be remembered, articulated, and reconstructed. It is a matter of choice. Could it even be a matter of survival?

Katherine Lang. Fragmented thinking

"I'm thirty-three now and up until I was twenty-five I would have said that I had too many other things to do. It seemed, too, that the women that I knew who had children were in a disadvantaged position a lot of the time. As mothers, it seemed that all of a sudden their power or influence had really changed in society generally, as well as their relationships with their husbands." She talks about her friends who, once they had children and became deeply involved in their children's lives, "changed what they wanted to do and what they were able to do with their own lives."

The decision to have a child was for Katherine "a long time brewing." At one time she even thought that she might not want to have children. "But," she says, speaking so quietly that I could barely hear, "I just didn't want to say that, because it doesn't even sound nice to say something like that. However, it was something I thought about. I was making this decision about me, my body, and my life, and that was the way it was. But between twenty-five to twenty-seven, it was almost a biological thing, a real physical kind of feeling, and I know that sounds kind of hokey, but it was that my periods were something that were making me think—each month my periods demonstrated that nothing had been done about that."

Eventually the time was right for her. "I had a really strong feeling before I missed my period. It happened to be a particular, *that* particular cycle that we had had lots of good sex, and there was a change in my body—like I knew. I could feel the change in my breasts, a real change, and then I missed my period. It made a difference. We went out for dinner and had wine with everybody else, and just because I had that feeling in me, that hunch, then obviously I couldn't, I shouldn't be drinking now. It would be an inappropriate thing to do." Katherine kept the glass of wine in front of her because she did not want anyone to suspect her pregnancy. She did not drink the wine.

Katherine's baby was born by cesarean section. Katherine's membranes ruptured, but her cervix only dilated four centimeters after a couple of days of labor. The surgery took place one stormy night a few days before Christmas. "And then when I was back in the room in the bed and people were attending me, cleaning up, taking blood pressure, and all this fuss and bother, Mike came in to see me and Mike told me that we'd had a girl and that she was eight pounds ten ounces. Mike said, 'You can see the baby if you want,' and I said, 'I can't.' I just didn't have the energy." Katherine did not see her daughter until the next morning. "When I first saw her I was really surprised at what she looked like. I didn't know what to expect—I guess I expected a fair child, she is dark, and I didn't expect such a big baby. Her face and her big chubby cheeks were really a surprise. I think that probably the real feeling of mothering happened over that first day. At first I think I was just too curious. I just looked at her as an object to examine and to see that all was there. But then, after a while, just being able to comfort her . . . that is, if I talked to her, she seemed to be soothed. She seemed to know somebody was there. When you get a response from the child to something that you're doing, that feels motherly then. Maybe that is when you start feeling it."

"I pricked Brett with a pin a couple of days ago," confesses Katherine when the baby is about two months old. "It was terrible. I was morose the whole afternoon. I felt so bad!" It took Brett a while to react and for Katherine to realize what had happened. "She finally did settle down and went to sleep, exhausted from crying, and I couldn't wait for her to wake up again so I could hold her and say, 'It's okay, I'm sorry.' When I think about the cesarean I wonder why—why it went that way, what was I doing or what was I not doing? Again, it is kind of a guilt thing. As I say, I've apologized to her, I don't know how many times—'I'm sorry, kid, that it happened like that.' I am trying to find out more about it from John [the doctor]. I want to know what the obstetrician wrote. I want to know why it was necessary to do it. I want to know her Apgar score. Perhaps there is a little bit of sadness that it happened that way, and there is a real sense, when you have a cesarean, of the inadequacy of your body. It didn't work right!

"I've got Brett on my mind all the time, whatever I am planning to do. It's ongoing. It's fragmented my thinking. For example, if I am watching the news and she is awake, I can't pay really good attention—or when I am on the phone. If she needs me for whatever reason, or if I am aware of her, other things have to go. I guess I think that mothers live a very fragmented existence."

Katherine talks of going back to work in the fall. In addition to thinking about the childcare arrangements and how she will work and still spend enough time with her baby, she also wonders how having a baby will affect her work, "because I have a baby at home who has more priority than the job." Yet she wonders, "You never get paid in money—that is, with any official recognition—for what you do as a mother.

And you do a lot. I don't want to think of it like work because it is all tied up in loving your baby, loving and caring for your baby. Perhaps there has got to be enough intrinsic reinforcement of what you are doing, or things may just get out of focus. I can't feel too strongly about that right now, but I sure can see how it might happen, that you start feeling, 'Why did I buy into this one?' "

Before Brett's birth, Katherine talks self-assuredly about her plans for the birth and her child. She plans her life carefully, it seems, like finding work to support her while she raises her child. She is independent, a woman who does things her own way. She has strong opinions on how she would like to give birth, based on research, reading, and talking with others. But in living with Brett, through pregnancy, the birth, and the first few weeks, Katherine begins to doubt. She begins to question herself, her decisions, her actions, like she "should not drink wine now." Before the birth she thought that a cesarean birth would not be a problem in the establishment of a good relationship with the baby, "because the relationship starts in pregnancy." She says, "It may be that a cesarean section is a kind of interruption in that relationship, but I think you can establish a good, if not better, relationship with your child afterwards." Yet, after the birth, she seems less sure. She apologizes to her baby for the birth: "I'm sorry that it happened like that." For Katherine, motherhood is full of guilt. "You feel guilty about a whole bunch of things—you are responsible for so many things and it is impossible to be one hundred percent on top of them all." The baby crying, not sleeping, being gassy, being hurt by a pin, dressed the wrong way, or being born by surgery triggers these uncomfortable guilt feelings. "What am I doing that's causing this to be like this?" She says, "I shouldn't have done that. Maybe it was the pizza." In Katherine's words we hear the tension between the need to be selfless and identified only by one's relationship (I am Brett's mother), and the need to be for the self and identified as oneself and one's relationship (I am Katherine and Brett is my daughter). Mothering is the living out of a tension between being for the self and being for the child. In order to remove the accusation of guilt one needs a more explicit articulation of the tension.

Katherine's talk shows how mothers are pulled toward the child and feel that they are responsible for everything that happens to their child. Many women who mother experience these same feelings. Judy Chicago in *The Birth Project* notes that although things like a miscarriage, abruptio placenta, or a deformed child are out of women's control, many women say, "I felt it was somehow my fault" (1985: 76). To have a child is to put oneself in question—involving inner change in a woman's understanding of herself. In commenting on the change, one mother says that her daughter has "forced me to confront dark places in my own soul—my desire to possess, to own; selfishness, or egocentricity; real doubts about the purity of my past loves, past actions" (Dowrick and Grundberg 1980: 79). In caring for the vulnerable, helpless, dependent, crying infant, mothers tend to look at themselves as the cause—even if what is happening is not in their immediate control. "Ariel is a great teacher. Not only does he force me to *see* my limitations; he has me—kicking and screaming—accepting them. For the first time in my life, I'm learning about love . . . about what it takes to nourish, maintain human life" (Chesler 1979: 191). In living with the child, women learn more about themselves and the mutuality of the mothering relation. They learn, too, to accept their own dark side, their limitations, mistakes, and egocentricity.

Although Katherine describes self-doubt and self-questioning as guilt, it may be more useful to understand these self-questionings as a positive impulse, a positive decentering of the self for the sake of the Other. Katherine says the pull of the child leads to fragmented thinking, which—instead of being negative—could be viewed as a way of thinking that moves from self to child and back to a self that is more reflective, more conscious of the reality of living with the child and with others. Fragmented thinking can be understood as the way a woman opens herself to her child and yet is true to herself, and is also constantly vigilant of both her child and herself. By creating space in the mother's body for her child, by creating space in her life for herself, by stretching her mind and stretching her body, mothering becomes a positive, complex, relational experience.

The negative effect of being fragmented also comes through in Katherine's self-questioning—expecting to be perfect, to meet all the child's needs, to do it right. We hear Katherine's own ambivalence: "Why did I buy into this one?" Although she loves her child and wants to be there for her, she seems caught in an expectation that mothering is a completely selfless, altruistic act, and that she must be perfect. Just as Katherine apologizes to Brett, perhaps we, communally, need to apologize to Katherine. How do we, communally, let Katherine down? Do cultural expectations induce her to see menstruation as a visible reminder of failing to do something about mothering? Are there expectations urging her to see cesarean birth as neither significant nor important for her? Or, perhaps, too important for her? Is there a difference between feeling guilty and feeling sad about having a cesarean birth? Is she doubly fragmented, perhaps? Is she fragmented in a positive way by the love for her child, and in a negative way by living in a society that often does not give concrete public value to that love and commitment? Why do women lose their influence and power in society when they become mothers? Society needs to think about how to support mothers. How do we assist the mother to work through her feelings about the cesarean birth, the fact that she had pizza, or that she unintentionally pricked her child? Does a mother's self-doubt about issues beyond her control relate to her position in society? How can women be supported through the experiences of infertility, adoption, or placing a child? How can we support the young single woman who chooses to live with her child?

How can we give more value to mothering? How can community support for the mothering relation be strengthened?

The situation of women in patriarchal societies complicates the valuing of the mothering relation. Women are the *other*—like Blacks, the aged, and the poor. But here the notion of "other" is not that of the relational Other, the child. When female writers—from Simone de Beauvoir to Mary Daly, from Adrienne Rich to Mary O'Brien—speak of women as *other*, they remind us that women live in a world focused on the norm of the male body (not subject to the cyclical nature of menstruation), the male-dominated public decision-making bureaucracy (which venerates objectivity, management, control, and efficiency), and the male-dominated healthcare establishment (where men hold most of the prestigious and powerful positions). The relational nature of mothering is given second place in such a world.

In the present economic, political, and social situation, many women responding to the child find that the relational commitment can be either empowering or disenfranchising, and in fact is often both. For at the same time as a woman may feel blessed by having a child in her life, by the very fact that she is a mother or is becoming a mother, she may be further oppressed. (Think of the single teenage mother who gets called a slut just for being pregnant.) Poverty, lack of employment opportunities, lack of parenting support services—such as flexible work hours and high-quality funded childcare—lack of support for mothers who stay at home full-time and for those who work outside of the home, and lack of financial assistance to keep good and healthy food on the table make the endless tasks that are involved in caring for the young child extremely difficult. So while women move toward a responsibility for the child (in their responsiveness to the positive Other), they are continually faced with the reality of their own *otherness* (a negative reality) in patriarchal culture.

In mothering a woman's focus becomes divided between responsibility for the baby and responsibility for herself. Should not both be considered? What is best for the baby cannot be overlooked, but what is good for the woman must also be kept in mind. I am reminded of a logo used on a newsletter about parenting and breastfeeding, where the baby was a silhouette in bright pink and the surrounding mother was colored in shadowy grey. In a societal effort to see the baby as central, there is the danger of the woman, the mother, losing herself—becoming a shadowy grey. In reality, however, the distinction between the experience of the mother and the responsibility of mother to child becomes blurred, especially when the child is a baby (Kathleen Sullivan, personal communication, October 1994). No longer is it just the woman or just the child who needs care; it is the mothering relation that needs to be attended to—a relation that affects us all, away from the self-centered concerns of "me, me, me" that Gwen Reid (an adopting mother) speaks about, and toward loving relations such as "telling my grandmother I love her," which Lorrie Newton (a placing mother) describes. Think, too, of Jasmine Jonson (a teen mother), who for the sake of her child stopped smoking, doing drugs, drinking alcohol, stayed home at night, and went back to school.

The turn from guilt to responsiveness does not necessarily mean that the woman who mothers loses herself. She realizes that to be *for* another, *with* another, means a conscious attention to the self; "Who am I?" and "What can I do?" Mothering is a relation, not a job. As Rachel, a teen mother, says, "Mothering is not babysitting." Mothering is a way of being, a relation that transcends all jobs, careers, divorces, and other relationships. As such it is worthy of particular attention and support. In saying that being a mother is not a job, I am not diminishing the work that mothers do in the everyday care of the children, especially the mothers who shoulder the full childcare responsibility. I am, rather, making an appeal for public regard for what it means for women to be mothers and workers, inside and outside the home, at the same time. Christiane Northrup in her 1994 book *Women's Bodies, Women's Wisdom* says, "once a woman has a baby, that child is a part of her twenty-four hours a day in ways that no one can explain until it happens to her. I was not prepared for the ache in my heart that occurred when I left my baby to go to work every day" (1994: xxiii–xxiv). For a mother to have a child on her mind means that the commitment to the child is always there. For many mothers this is their primary commitment, and it needs to be supported and fostered in the public world. How is the mothering relation learned? How can it be supported and made stronger? The relation of mother and child, so vividly experienced in the body during pregnancy, birth, nursing, and nurturance, must always be understood in the reality of a particular culture, a particular milieu. "Mother love is anything other than natural and instead represents a matrix of images, meanings, sentiments, and practices that are everywhere socially and culturally produced" (Scheper-Hughes 1992: 341).

THE TURN TO THE CHILD

How does a woman become responsive to the child? How does a woman come to live as mother—for her child—and yet for herself? Does it mean that a woman gives her body completely over to the care of others during pregnancy? Does it mean that a woman's own experience of giving birth is secondary to the experience of birth for the child? Does it mean that a woman should stop her own projects and devote herself to the care of her child full-time? Does it mean that a woman should stop being in relation to other adults on a daily basis?

In mothering, the turn toward the child is learned first and foremost in the body. By "learned in the body" I mean that it is learned in the lived body of a woman who lives in a particular space and time, in a particular social and cultural context. The way of the mother is learned bodily, socially, and cognitively, at the same time. The competing claims of *biological* versus *cultural* lose the exclusiveness that these positions suggest. As the mother turns toward her child through pregnancy, birth, and nurturance, the boundaries (social as well as physical) between mother and child lose their sharp definitions, at least for a while.

Pregnancy

The experience of carrying a fetus within one's body is hard to explain or even to describe. How does one experience being tied to another, a very dependent being, in such an intimate, deep way? Women can and do talk about this experience—the experience of the embodied presence of the fetus, and the experience of becoming present to the fetus, that is, being attentive to the new being as it develops. It is hard for rational minds to understand what is not easily or concretely ordered, such as this embodied experience of knowing the fetus to be a part of oneself and yet not oneself. A male friend—rather carelessly, I thought—remarked how disgusting it must be to have a baby inside. He used words like "gross" and "awful." The experience of holding a baby within one's body is something that men cannot truly fathom. Yet many men, unlike my friend, have some sense of the mystery and awe in this experience. For women, the wonder and pleasure (as well as the discomfort and pain) of the experience speaks of a remarkable intimacy. For women this experience is, indeed, awe-ful, full of awe. This exceptional interrelationship has been described by Kathryn Rabuzzi as a "kind of interactive, two-in-one-self," where the selfhood of the woman becomes "motherselfhood" (1988: 43, 52). Strange, yes—a relationship of intimate, involved participants, and a relationship that causes growth and change in both. Pregnancy is often seen primarily as a physical state, easily observed in the woman and now, through ultrasound, observed in the fetus as well. To be pregnant refers to the experience of carrying a child in the womb, but pregnant also means creative, brimming with significance, ready to give birth to something—an idea, an inspiration.

The pregnancy experience, as a human experience, is part of the natural world (the physical body) and the social world (the community) at the same time (Braine and Lesser 1988). Of course, a woman's pregnant body can be easily objectified, analyzed, and treated abstractly, as vividly illustrated in the technology of obstetrics. The woman's embodied experience of giving birth to her baby, however, placed concretely within her family, friends, and social community, is not easily articulated. Giving birth to a child, creating a new life, must not be isolated and treated in a technical way as a problem to be managed. Rather, giving birth to a child gives the community (us) the opportunity to renew itself, to begin again. Giving birth to a child means brimming with significance for the family and the community.

Pregnancy is often seen as being for the baby; yet, pregnancy also involves the growth of a woman through her body and through her thoughts and emotions. The woman is not merely a vessel for the use of this other developing being. She, too, is developing and changing. It is not insignificant that in a recent news report of heart surgery performed while the fetus was in the uterus there is no mention of the mother—just "mother's womb" and "mother's skin" (*The Edmonton Journal*, February 1, 1990). As we more frequently take a technological look at the woman and fetus as separate entities, it becomes credible for the fetus to become the patient and for the woman to be seen as a human incubator. From the point of view of women's experience of pregnancy such notions are totally foreign, in fact, repugnant. Pregnancy is not experienced as one versus the other (that is, one plus one); rather, it is one with the other (two in one)—an altogether different relationship. The technological world of medicine does not understand this distinction. Technological fragmentation easily separates woman and fetus, biology and culture, private and public, mother and child—and in doing so easily destroys, or at least disregards, the relational impulse.

While the fetus grows and develops into human form (and it is important to remember that this cannot happen without the woman), the woman changes into a mother (which cannot happen without a child). She changes not only in her body, but, as we have seen, in her very nature, her way of seeing the world, her relationships, and her thinking. The talk of women during pregnancy centers on this changing understanding of the self— "Who am I?"—through the recognition of the fetus/baby—"Who are You?" Over the nine months, both of these themes take on new meanings for the woman. As a woman begins to recognize the reality of the child, she is also attentive to her self. In this experience, being attentive to the baby is not a *disengagement* of the self, but an understanding of the *engagement* of mother with child. The process of engagement with the child cannot be divided into distinct stages, but has a number of attributes, which will differ with each mother's experience.

This Is My Body: The Idea of the Baby. On first recognition of pregnancy, the sense of the baby is distant. A woman may say "I am going to have a baby," but the baby is just an idea, perhaps even a secret for a while, something that a woman may hold close to her heart—like Glenda Richards, who wants "just to get used to the idea, and just sort out how we feel about it and adjust to it before we share it with anybody else." Or Sylvie Foster, who says, "It was mine, a secret, it was something I had." Later one would share the fact of the pregnancy and the "going to have a baby" with others: husband, family, and friends. The baby, as an idea or an abstraction, seems more true for the father than for the mother. Women wait for the inner signs (movement, heartbeat) or the outer signs (the tighter skirts, etc.) to make them realize that there indeed is a fetus/child present, whereas men could make the baby an object without waiting for signs within themselves. For example, Nancy Thompson suggests that if abnormalities were discovered through the amniocentesis, Peter (her husband) would be "more comfortable with the notion of aborting than she would be." Also, the father can more easily talk to "the baby," whereas the mother can only talk to the baby inwardly, as "a part of herself." Recall how Michelle Freeman (a teen mother) describes how during pregnancy her boyfriend could easily talk of giving up the baby for adoption, while for her "the kid's sitting there kicking me in the stomach." Perhaps it is easier for men to imagine the baby, to think concretely of a baby as a separate being, while women are tied to experiencing the baby through their own bodies.

For the woman, the idea of the baby is tied to what is happening to her: bodily changes that are often uncomfortable ("perhaps I am just sick"); a growing body ("maybe it is just fat"); feeling vulnerable about being faced with overwhelming tasks; and the fear that "I, myself, will be lost in the process and will not have control of my life." Nancy describes pregnancy as a world where you are not in charge any more. For her, pregnancy is an experience where "suddenly, because your placenta is pumping out all these hormones, your life is changed. You feel lousy and it's not like you can just put on a stiff upper lip and carry on. It wasn't possible. What I had planned to do just had to go by the board. And that bothered me a lot." The focus of a woman during the experience of pregnancy is primarily on the self, "how I am feeling, how I can handle this new experience. I need friends and family to care for me, I fear losing myself, I fear losing control, and becoming dependent on others." The idea of the baby is found in the words "It is my body—Is there really a baby in there?" The woman has not yet begun, in a bodily way, to recognize the reality of the baby.

This Is My Body and My Baby. The first encounter with the fetus comes through hearing the heartbeat, seeing the ultrasound, and feeling a movement. "I think once it started to really move I started to identify that it was a baby, not just something happening to me," says Nancy. These profound stirrings indicate a recognition that there is someone else there. For Sylvie, "Yes, now it is very real. Now I can think of the baby concretely. I have contact with this baby now where I didn't before. And now it is very real." Nancy explains, "I had ultrasound quite early. I saw the heart beating and that was wonderful for me. Although I had sore breasts and felt morning sickness, there was this nagging feeling that maybe I wasn't really pregnant after all. Maybe there wasn't anything in there, maybe I had just made up those symptoms. It was so nice to see the embryo at that point and the heart beating. It made it more real." The first encounters with the sound of the heartbeat and the picture of the moving fetus make women sense someone other than themselves. It is real. That is, pregnancy is real and the abstract baby is really there, but not yet as an individual: "The baby is not a separate being, but an extension of myself."

During the period of pregnancy when the baby becomes more *real*, women plan for the baby in terms of space and supplies needed (not necessarily doing anything), discuss these plans with others, and discuss with partners (and/or other important people in their lives) how this coming baby will change relationships. There is concern that the coming baby can diminish the relationship between partners. Talking with others seems to be significant—women talk about being let into a secret club, a club that consists of women who have children. Nancy mentions how Peter is also allowed into a self-help group of men who tell him what to expect, not only during the pregnancy, but after the birth.

This Is My Body: This Is My Baby. Sylvie starts to see the beginnings of the individual child through the following event.

It definitely has a life of its own. I had been reading on my side, and then I turned on my back and the baby didn't like that position. I told Bob I could feel it tensing and doing things, and then it started moving. It had these deliberate movements. And, as for me, I knew that somebody else was in there. It was a somebody who could decide when it wants to do something. All the other things were smaller pushes but this was a deliberate turning over and pushing and getting more space. It was definitely someone separate. Bob saw it too.

Women make guesses about what the movements mean. Nancy remarks, "Sometimes I think he moves just to move, so I don't always interpret it as a sign that he's uncomfortable." They find satisfaction in making sense of the behavior, the movements, and responses of the fetus. They think about the characteristics of their child. The encounters with the fetus remind Glenda that "before it was me, but it's not any more, this is my baby, I really feel *somebody*." The coming to know the individual child continues to develop through play, through the movement, toward a more distinct recognition that this fetus/baby is a separate/separating being. "When it definitely feels like a separate being is when it makes its presence known in an uncomfortable way." Sylvie continues, "I talk to it after it's been punching and making me very uncomfortable, and then I realize it's a whole, separate, uncomfortable person in there because it is tossing and turning and poking me, and I realize that that's the separate baby—but while it is in me, it's two of us sharing this body, so I tell the baby to take mind of that and share." Sylvie asks her baby to be fair. We hear attention to both the needs of the self (the woman) and the needs of the Other (the fetus). In all relationships, not just that of mother and child, there must be attention to the needs of both partners in the relationship. In mothering, however, there seems to be a ready-made rule that says that the needs of the child always come first. Such a rule needs qualification and reconsideration. The child's needs are important, but if there is no attention to the needs of the mother as well, both child and mother will suffer (Swigart 1991).

In talking to the baby within and shifting to make room for him or her ("he reminds me to sit up"), mothers recognize that this baby is someone, someone who is strong and vigorous, and who, as Sylvie says, "makes its own mind to do gymnastics and punch around." The woman can hold the baby by wrapping her arms around her own belly, push back on a foot that is pushing too hard, or talk back and forth to him or her in a playful way. This talking to the baby, this giving and taking that often begins before birth, leads women to think about the actual separation, when she will meet the biologically independent child. As the fetus/baby gets bigger, women can begin to imagine pushing the baby out and prepare for that separation. Some women, like Sylvie, say they expect pain as a necessary part of their separation from their child. Sylvie believes that "the pain is a mark of rite of passage, you know, that it's necessary. All the major events in your life you have to go through with a bit of pain. And I hope I feel some. I don't want it *that* easy." Glenda thinks that "the pain and the labor and what you go through really can affect mentally how I feel about the baby becoming a separate identity, apart from myself. I think the pain of labor, what is going to happen in labor, is going to be necessary for me to accept the separation." It is through the pain of labor that the woman comes to see the child face to face.

In exploring the changing attention to both the self (the mother) and the other (the baby), it is important to recognize that these processes do not occur at a particular time in pregnancy. Sometimes, as noted in discussion of the placing mother, the woman's recognition of the baby as a person does not happen until after the birth. Recall Sally Corbett saying, "Before I held him, he was just a ball in my belly, and it didn't really mean as much." But the first time she held him Sally felt that she could not place her child. The child had become a person to her. As the mother experiences herself *with* child, she becomes ready to take on the responsibility to be *for* the child. Now Sally thinks again about placing her child with the adopting parents she has chosen. She experiences her responsibility and the relationship to her child differently.

The birth itself shows how the relationship of mother and child continues to include other family members—the father, the grandparents, and friends. The birth is an extension of the relation begun before birth, and from that perspective it becomes more than the birth of the child. It becomes the birth of the family and a renewal of community. B. Joan Lawrence tells the story of her granddaughter's birth. She says of her laboring daughter, "She is strong. She is beautiful in her labour. Her body, mind, and spirit are working together at all times for the good of herself and her child and family and her community and the future of the world" (Lawrence 1996).

The First Breath

Then the family stills to view one of the truly astonishing wonders of life: the first breath. As Jonathan takes his first gulp of oxygen, his complexion slowly warms from an eerie blue to a glowing pink. . . . The joy of the family is palpable. They fuss. They adore. They coo. Jonathan responds . . . he is wide-eyed—lies serene in his mother's arms. (McRoberts 1984: B9)

This description of a baby's first breath was written by a newspaper reporter who attended a birth. Here is another description of the first breath, as witnessed by a father. He writes, "Ella was born. We put our hands on her head, we caressed the warm, moist body, and felt her chest expand with the first breath of life, and then heard her let out her first cry" (Russell Kelly, personal communication, June 1987). Others describe the first breath differently. A respected obstetrician, an advocate for the use of fetal monitors with all laboring women, agrees that the first minutes of the life of a newborn infant are most important. "But," he says, "it is not in the dim light in the delivery room [referring here to the Leboyer's method] . . or . . . early skin contact [in reference to the work of Klaus and Kennell] . . . but [it is] warmth, a normal Apgar score, and a high umbilical cord pH which are really important (Baumgarten 1981: 271).

While the last voice may be said to express an objective view and the first two may be seen as subjective, possibly romantic views, the language they use displays opposing views of the baby's first breath. It is not, however, just a matter of language; rather, language points to the whole context in which the baby takes that first breath. In each situation what is sought is a healthy baby and mother, but divergent forms of knowledge are used to achieve that outcome. In the views of the reporter and the father, we see an outcome encompassing a respect for the wonder of a new life (that independent breath), the response of the family (warm caresses, palpable joy), the response of the baby (change in color, wide-eyed, serene, the first cry) in the arms of the family—the focus is on the relation. The obstetrician's account—with the goals of environmental warmth (possibly a warm blanket, an incubator, or the woman's belly), a normal Apgar score (an evaluation of the baby's heart rate, respiratory effort, muscle tone, reflex irritability, and color), and a high umbilical cord pH (a blood sample taken from the cord)—has lost all traces of Jonathan or Ella, or any baby, the mother, the family, and even, perhaps, respect for the wonder of life. In the last account the birth has become a homogenous, technological experience (Stolte 1990). The obstetrician's words ring clearly of the absence of relation; the focus is on the body of the child as an object. The first experience of the baby in the obstetric view is one of measurement and calculation. How well does the baby measure up?

In *Hard Choices: Mixed Blessings of Modern Technology*, a book by B. D. Colen (1986), the stories of parents with children whose lives are saved by medical expertise bring attention to dilemmas created by separating the technological and the social. The following story tells of parents' experiences with their child, who was initially salvaged (a word that is often used) at birth through technological expertise. In this passage the father is talking. He says, "I got fixated on all the numbers. . . . Is the last significant digit really a significant digit? It usually turned out the answer was no. I got fixated on that, but the baby was responsive. That seemed wonderful to me. You scratched its feet, and it would kick its feet. It would grab your finger, not like a real infant, but it would definitely curl its fingers around the finger." He then describes how the mother, who developed infection following the very difficult cesarean birth, was finally allowed out of isolation to see her child for the first time. "When she [the mother] came down and talked to her, she [the baby] opened her eyes for the first time. . . . When my wife started talking to her and touching her, her absorption of oxygen went up. . . . It turned out later that whenever either one of us spoke to her and touched her at the same time, we could see her respond by her blood oxygen going up" (Colen 1986: 133). Notice, again, the language. When the father talks about his child in relation to the machines and numbers, he refers to the baby as *it*, but when he talks about himself and his wife talking to their child, it is *her*. Notice, too, the impact of touch—the blood oxygen would go up. Talk and touch made a difference.

In our present birth environments in Western culture, we take the technological approach for granted. It is the norm. Even the birthing rooms (the places in which "normal" births take place) are equipped with all the latest technological machines—the fetal monitor, the intravenous supplies, the suction apparatus, the respirator, the incubator, scales, test tubes—however well they may be hidden behind the colorful curtains and wallpaper, the new oak bed, the comfortable chair, the TV, and the telephone. Of course, the Apgar score is a valued tool, giving an important assessment of the baby's functions, and the cord pH does give clues about dangerous chemical imbalances. Yet, we must remind ourselves that technology is not neutral, and as we surround ourselves with the taken-for-granted technological influence we need to consider how technology mediates the experience for the baby and for the mother. I have explored more fully the woman's experience of the fetal monitor in a paper (Kelpin 1985) that exposes the impact of amplifying certain information while reducing or not attending to other information.

Let us go back to the baby's first breath. This time, it is seen through the eyes of a grandmother, Regina Hobbs, who was present at the birth of her daughter Anna's second baby girl, Alexandra—a sister for Jena.

Regina Hobbs. Positive anger

"And then the baby came. And the first thing I heard, 'it's a girl.' And we looked and this little girl won't breathe. I thought to myself, 'It's OK, Anna, you can have another one'—that went through my mind. 'It's OK,' I didn't say it, I just felt it. And then I thought, 'Don't do that to my daughter. She worked so hard for you for nine months, and worked for hours and hours—don't do that to her.' I felt really angry with the baby, for not breathing and giving Anna such a rough time. I couldn't get rid of that feeling until the next morning, and I had to have a cry on somebody's shoulder.

"It was so scary. They massaged the baby and moved her legs, gave the baby oxygen, did mouth-to-mouth. And Anna kept saying, 'Come on, little one.' 'Come on, little one.' 'Come on, little one.' The heart was always beating and that was a good thing. The critical moment for Alexandra was when the midwives put her on Anna's tummy after she had caught herself [had taken a breath] not really rhythmic, yet—put on Anna's tummy and then she got her color and that was it.

"Sure it was a traumatic and scary moment for all of us, and we felt we were all a part of giving life to this little one—even if it meant being angry with her. As a matter of fact, talking about it now, I understand the positive part of the anger. I didn't before, I felt guilty for being angry."

The ambulance was called, but in the few minutes it took to come, the baby responded, took her first breath. After assessing the situation, the ambulance attendant was pleased to see what was happening—because of his own experience. Apparently, his first-born baby had trouble breathing, and was taken immediately to the neonatal intensive care unit, and for two hours the mother and father were in agony because they couldn't be with the baby. "And of course," Regina continues, "the baby had the same experience."

Yet, what is the baby's experience? Can we know for sure? When I requested that my daughter remain with me at birth, I recall being told that "babies like it wrapped in a blanket in the nursery." Do they? Is that what they are longing for? Bollnow claims, "we can understand the child only from the standpoint of the adult and never the inverse" (1987: 42). How, then, do we understand? Is it important to understand? What is it like to be in the world as a child? Maybe the question should rather be, how do we respond to the child as a child, as a social being? Can we imagine what a child needs?

The Kangaroo Method, a program incorporating skin-to-skin holding of the premature baby by the mother or father, is being introduced in many neonatal intensive care facilities in Europe and North America (See Gale, Fanck, and Lund 1993; Victor and Persoon 1994). This program, developed in Colombia by a nurse researcher, Vivian Wahlberg, and others, arose out of severe economic constraints, problems with cross-infection, high mortality and morbidity rates, and parental abandonment, and is based on a deep respect for the natural relation between mothers and babies. In this program, mothers breastfeed their premature infants as often as necessary to keep them satisfied and keep them warm by carrying them skin-to-skin in an upright position between their breasts. The initial results are favorable. A premature baby born at thirty-two weeks' gestation, weighing 1,850 grams, was breastfed eight hours after birth, lost no weight in the first twenty-four hours, and was discharged at thirty-six hours. It appears that she is developing normally. Reductions in mortality, morbidity, and parental abandonment have been observed with this program, which is a radical approach considering current Western practices in the care of the premature infant. "Reflection upon these improvements led to the realization that the maternal milieu—warmth, nourishment and love—does indeed provide the ideal environment for premature infants" (Anderson, Marks, and Wahlberg 1986: 808). Lauren Wyman says she feels magic in holding her tiny premature son against her breast, and has no doubt that he too is pleasured by this close touch, for "when they came to take him away, he didn't want to let go" (Keating 1994: 23). Here the mother-child relation is nurtured. We learn from the kangaroo.

We also learn from Jane Gibson, who took the time to experience the first look of her daughter at birth and to return it. We hear the power of that look as Jane says, "you can't turn her down." We know that infants, within minutes of birth, visually follow a face-like pattern, and that mothers are interested in making eye contact (Lozoff, Brittenham, Trause, Kennell, and Klaus 1977), yet we need to attend to what actually happens. What is the significance of eye contact? As we exchange looks with the child—our child—we cannot hide ourselves, and may come to know our responsibility and accept it. Perhaps, as we return the look of the child—of Lisa, of Jonathan, of Ella, of Jena, of Alexandra—we are required to question ourselves, and in doing so we learn what we must be and do. Perhaps it takes a certain kind of looking, of anger, of listening, of waiting, of responding—which reveals a profound respect for the new being that comes into this world. The respect that Robin Dillon (1992) talks of is respect that is attentive to the particularity of the person, the person as he or she is. Dillon's notion of respect, which she calls care respect, transcends the Kantian abstract notion of *person as such* to focus on the *human being as herself.* "Care respect responds to persons both in the richness of this distinguishing detail and in the shared humanity that encompasses and is encompassed in it" (Dillon 1992: 119).

Regina Hobbs, the grandmother who spoke of her anger, is also a hospital chaplain. From her experience in intensive care units with the dying elderly she comments: "Because we institutionalize birth and institutionalize death we are really losing touch with real life, losing touch with ourselves really. We find birth too bloody, and we find dying too horrible, yet without birth and death there is no life." Mae Stolte, a psychoanalyst, agrees that when one separates spirit and matter, as occurs in most Western births, the experience becomes one-sided and incomplete, "depriving us of the energy that is inherent in the birth process" (1990: 7). The spirit energy felt in the baby's first breath can transform those who watch and support: Each birth of a child offers us a magic that helps us to live. The birth of a baby is a quickening of our social and cultural life—it awakens us to our moral commitments to the child and to each other. It triggers the impulse to be moral.

I have explored the bodily and socially constructed experience of pregnancy and birth, in which the birth mother and her family move toward the child—to be with and for the child. In the next section I will focus on nurturance, which, too, is both bodily and socially experienced.

Nurturance

"I guess I started to feel motherly when she responded to something I did—if I talked to her, she seemed to quiet, seemed to know I was there and able to comfort her," says Katherine Lang. The ability of women to nourish is something to be cherished. It is important to the child and to the mother, it ties a mother to her child in necessary ways. The most pristine image of nurturance one can think of is a mother nursing her child. The mother and child are comfortably meshed together in an experience of mutual participation and interaction. Domination of one over the other does not fit into this picture. From the Indo-European root *sneu*, to nurture means to suckle and to flow (Morris 1975)—that is, one cannot have one without the other, one needs a giver as well as a receiver. Although one might at first glance think it is obvious that the mother is the giver and the child the receiver, this notion is not absolutely clear. While the mother *gives* her milk to her child, the child *takes* the milk from the mother. While the suck of the child causes the milk to be produced and flow, it is the presence of the mother that stimulates the action of the infant to suckle. As the baby receives milk, the mother receives comfort and physical well-being. The image of breastfeeding as nurturance shows giving and receiving as concrete and embodied, interactive and engaged; it is an activity where more giving (suckling) produces more replenishment (flowing). Neumann (1955) describes the woman's third archetypal transformation as the transformation of blood into milk. Here milk is symbolic of the outpouring actions "to nourish and protect, to keep warm and hold fast"—actions done for the sake of the child. The symbols that belong to the image of the breast are open in character— the bowl, the goblet, the cup, and the Grail—and accentuate the giving, protecting, warming aspect of the feminine archetype of nourishment.

But nurturance is not confined to the breastfeeding woman. Women nurture their babies in many ways, such as bottlefeeding, holding close, singing, and rocking. Yet we can learn from those bodily experiences we sometimes label "natural." I remember a particular episode when it was me and my baby who needed care and nurturance. It was a summer afternoon, late, just before supper. My son was still very young—no more than a week or two. He was frantically trying to settle into nursing on my right breast, frantically attempting to latch onto my nipple. You might imagine what he was doing—getting more and more frustrated and demanding, more and more agitated. I was getting more and more frustrated, and more and more agitated, too. We were both crying. I remember finally giving up and taking my baby outside to his father, who was overhauling the motor on our car. "Here, I can't do it," I wept. Much to his credit, my husband gathered us up, took us back into the house, sat me with Sem in our rocking chair, made us as comfortable as possible, probably got me a beer, and played the guitar until my baby and I slowly relaxed into the feeding—him suckling, me flowing, both feeling relieved and blessed. My husband nurtured us. We needed support. Sem and I, in our relation, needed relations with others.

The move to sharing the tasks of caring for the baby with others was discussed by many of the mothers I interviewed. Katherine talks about how she rushed home from shopping with thoughts of the child: "I felt it [in my breasts] if I was even just thinking about her. I would start to feel really full and kind of anxious to get home. I'd sometimes just forego doing something that I thought I would do, just to get home." Jane, too, remarks on the time it takes to really see the child as an independent person. "I left Lisa with Jim and I phoned when I got there fifteen minutes later, and then rushed home. The ties are incredible. The umbilical cord is not really cut for the first while. Now I can go out and not worry about her as much—I don't need her in my sight so much." Nel Henry, an adopting mother, says she had trouble leaving Timothy and at first left him only with family; even then she was not comfortable, for, she laughingly goes on, "I don't think anyone else could do as good a job as I can."

"While the primary interest of mothers, early on, is the preservation and nourishment of this new life, it is not long before other interests, such as fostering the child's growth, and shaping an acceptable child also become important" (Ruddick 1983: 219–223). These interests demand change on the part of the woman and involve moving away from the child. Weaning, substituting other food for breast milk, is one of the first experiences of letting go of the child. Moving away means feeling comfortable with someone else holding and soothing your baby while you go out to dinner, or with the child staying overnight with grandparents. Jane's admittance that she does not need Lisa in her sight so much may be an aspect of weaning—just like when Anna responds to people who remark on Jena's beauty by saying, "Yes, she is, isn't she?" rather than "Thank you." A mother's nurturing love respects the individuality of her child and the child's separateness from herself as the mother. At the same time, there is a realization that the mother's body and her attentive love hold an ongoing and lasting aspect of support for the child. The fact that the woman's body carries and nourishes the child ties a mother to her sons and daughters in a unique and intimate way. It does not mean, however, that birth mothers are alone in their giving of attentive love—other mothers (such as adopting mothers), fathers, and other relatives are also subject to the moral claim of the child.

I think again of my son. He was perhaps four weeks old—how hard it is to remember dates and times you once thought you would never forget. I was nursing him every three or four hours. I was tired and had lain down for a nap. After a long sleep, I woke refreshed. Suddenly, thoughts of my child rushed through my body—my breasts were painful and were starting to leak. But why had I not heard his cry? I was confused by this long sleep. I did not expect that I could have slept through his need for me. I found him in the garden contentedly sleeping in his carriage beside his father. His father had changed him and fed him with the breast milk that I had saved. Someone else could feed my baby! I was not always needed! My husband remembers that day, too. He found out that he could care for his child in a new way. Before that experience, his care had been for us as mother and child, as one. Now he had a glimpse of his unique and personal relationship with his child. He had fed him. It was a turning point for both of us.

Women nurture babies (bodily in breastfeeding), but even this so-called natural experience is culturally mediated. We are aware of the many ways a community supports (or does not support) "natural" experiences such as breastfeeding. Attachment and separation (holding fast and letting go) are in a dialectic relation. First, there is the intrauterine bond, followed by the separation of birth for the sake of the relation between mother and child; then there is the growing and maturing separation of mother and child for the sake of a deeper relational bond. Yet both forms of separation are not simply something the mother grants: the baby is born in its own time and grows at its own rate. The child gradually realizes adult freedom because the child wins it. As the child grows and moves away from the mother, and the mother lets the child go, both mother and child recognize more clearly the selfhood of each other.

Christine Martin, who from early pregnancy talks about her need to continue in her career, wants to be a good mother and still pursue her career. She says, "There is quite a bit of challenge in combining the two. It is sobering thinking about the future, about maintaining my career and my relationship to my child. And yet what I couldn't anticipate before was how important my child is to me and how strong that part of me is." In fact, her mothering influences her work, she says. "I can't switch off who I am with my child. He is too much a part of me. How I relate to my husband and my child is where I get my ideas." Of course, it is not always easy for Christine, since both she and her husband want to be parents and to have careers. Katherine Lang, in moving back to full-time work says to her boss, "I have too much to do." She would never have said that before. Before Brett was born, she would have come early or stayed late to get the work done. Now she is not prepared to do that. Her thoughts are directed to her child. She cannot ignore her relation, her response to her child.

The tension experienced by mothers who work outside of the home is felt in the tasks of being responsible to both child and work at the same time.

If instead of accusing the mother of being unreliable because of her competing claims, the work world supported the mother in her commitment to the child, that tension would be reduced. Instead of considering mothers' commitments to children as negative, the work world should consider the child when planning work schedules. As more fathers take on the daily responsibilities of children, negative attitudes to child commitments may change.

The problem of childcare is a real one in today's society. Some assert that there should be more and better daycare, even universal daycare. Others maintain that daycare cannot meet children's need to have at least one person care for them in *irrational* ways—ways made possible by unconditional love. While there are no perfect parents and no perfect homes, the best place for a child to gain the basic foundation of human life may be found within the home. But the reality of modern life has moved away from the possibility that one parent, often the mother, is able (financially, socially, or otherwise) to stay home with the child. Can we imagine a society where the care of children is a public commitment—a commitment that would include wonderful daycare facilities, support for women or men to stay at home without jeopardizing career choices and rewards, and truly flexible workdays that do not penalize workers, either part- or full-time?

The first task is to recognize and acknowledge the reality and value of mothering work. "Days are full of doing things," says Jane, "but nothing gets done." Life is unpredictable. Judy Chicago's image of the faceless lady as mother expresses the price women pay as nurturers, "as trapped by the needs of those one gives life to" (1985: 92, 96). Chronic fatigue, disorganization, multitudinous commitments, guilt, a fragmented existence all come with the nourishing requirements of the Other, the child. It was what Christine worried about before pregnancy, "You see, work is manageable, you know what you can do, you organize, while women who mother are fatigued and harassed and have trouble trying to accomplish all they need to do."

How does one organize time with a new baby? Even time, linear time, gets turned upside down. "They say to be there at eight," says Katherine, "so you try to be there by that time, which may not necessarily fit in with the way she would normally be doing things." "I think I am still organized to a degree, and I think about things ahead of time," Susan McLaren acknowledges, "but I start making dinner at two in the afternoon when he's settled down. I know that at supper time he is up. I just take advantage of the time I have." Even sex has its designated time: "If you want to have sex, we have to do it *now* because it is twenty to ten and the baby is asleep. Whatever happened to spontaneous lovemaking?" asks Christine. Instead of hours and minutes, work time, coffee time, or dinner time, the days are broken into sleep time, feeding time, bathing time, and laundry time. Time may seem endless, and one wonders if one can live through it. There is never enough time for sleep. There is not much time for oneself, as a mother.

How can one give more time to children? We hear about full-time mothers, part-time mothers, latchkey children, and even the notion of quality versus quantity time. In institutions built to care for children there is slotted time—going to the bathroom time, eating lunch time, cleaning up time, and so on, almost like the regimes of scientific mothering (a fragmenting of tasks). Where is the freedom of play time, doing nothing time, and private time that we all, especially children, need? How can we meet the needs of children and the needs of the mother?

There is danger in trivializing mother love by negating it, putting it down, and making it something private, which may not be valued in the public world. There is also danger in seeing mother love outside of the cultural, communal domain. From "a child only a mother could love," to the once-a-year accolades of Mother's Day, the love of the mother, the responsibility of motherhood, gets taken for granted as naturally woman's duty and sphere. In *Death Without Weeping*, Nancy Scheper-Hughes (1992) describes the world of Alto do Cruzeiro as a place where the ambiguities of mothering are intensely expressed, where neglect and intense attachment coexist. These Brazilian mothers, who turn away from certain ill-fated babies and abandon them to an early death, will in turn greet a baby who has shown a "hidden talent for life" with grateful joy and deep and lasting affection. The circumstances in this culture are such that mothers have to select which babies will get the limited resources available. Is this any different than mothers who refrain from connecting to the child they are adopting until they feel secure the child will stay with them? To be sure, the situation is different in degree, but is it different in kind? Once mothers feel confident that the child will be theirs, or will live with them, they give themselves to that connection, which becomes one of the most intense attachments.

Yet, mothering is attachment that needs a detachment, a holding close and letting go, at the same time. "To love a child without seizing or using it, to see the child's reality with the patient, loving eye of attention—such loving and attending might well describe the separation of mother and child from the mother's point of view" (Ruddick 1983: 224). To have a child on one's mind is a way of being and not merely an emotional reaction to children. Because "the passions of maternity are so sudden, intense, and confusing that women themselves often remain ignorant of the perspective, the thought, that is developed from mothering," says Sara Ruddick (1989: 10). Ruddick describes maternal thinking as an interplay between intellect and feeling, not primarily an emotional response. The way of the mother is a way of being and thinking about relations with children where the child is central. In order for mothers to give that centrality to children there is a need for real support. How can we create a world where all children will have mothers with the resources to mother them?

FREEDOM TO CHOOSE

The choice of whether or not we respond to the claim of a child—that is, whether or not we accept the relational commitment to the child—now needs our renewed attention. Response to the claim of the child is found within the choice to have children: in making the choice one opens oneself to the claim of the child. Reproductive knowledge abounds, making reproductive choice a real possibility for many women. Whether or not women are able to exercise choice has to do with cultural attitudes, power, resources, and respect for individuals—letting them judge their own suitability to have a child in their lives. One can decide against bringing a child into the world by celibacy, choosing the time of intercourse, contraception, and/or abortion. One can bring a child into the world by bodily conception, artificial insemination, or in vitro fertilization. One can adopt a child or place a child for adoption. One can raise a child even if unmarried and alone. Or one can choose not to have a child in one's life at all. Of course, we must be careful not to generalize this notion of choice. Some people have more ability to choose than others. Fiona Nelson (1995) warns that the ideology of reproductive choice has a dark underbelly—that we have been duped to think we have choice when, in fact, the conditions and requirements of mothering have not changed.

The biblical story of Adam, Eve, and the snake in the Garden of Eden is often seen as a story of the fall of humankind into sin. Another reading of the story, however, emphasizes the choice of freedom: "Then the Lord God said, 'Now the man has become like one of us, and has knowledge of what is good and what is bad' " (Genesis 3: 22, Today's English Version). Adam (the Hebrew word for mankind) and Eve (a name that sounds similar to the Hebrew word for life) in eating the fruit chose knowledge and freedom to make their own decisions about how to live. They chose to be with each other, to know each other, to desire each other, and to have children. The story of freedom is a story of relationship—life is about relations with one another, and about choice of how we act towards each other, choosing between what is good and what is bad (Chernin 1987).

In Western society there is a strong trend toward individualism, with emphasis on personal autonomy and attention to individual rights and self-determination. The relational impulse puts more emphasis on the connection between people than on their separateness. It is helpful to think of the distinction between the individual and the person: "An *individual* is defined by what distinguishes it from other individuals. . . . A *person* is defined by the relationship to others, to other persons and to other beings in general. We are born as individuals, but our task is to become persons"

(Capra and Steindl-Rast 1991: 95). Connections between people are important. It is through connections and relations that we come to know ourselves more fully as persons, a process that has no end. There is no way to definitely say, "Now, he or she is a person." Personhood is a process.

We have extensive knowledge about how to conceive and birth children and how to prevent the conception and birth of children. We can choose when and where to bring children into our lives. I propose that an understanding of the relational commitment between mother and child can guide moral responses to questions of how and when. I explore the abortion dilemma as an example of this moral commitment to the Other. Instead of getting caught in the rights debate (either pro-life or pro-choice), or the personhood debate (based on a theological, philosophical, or medical view), or the view that abortion is only a problem to be solved (with a technological solution), we need to turn our attention to the responsibility inherent in the relation between mother and child. From the point of view of the relational commitment, it is the woman herself who must struggle to know what is the right thing to do. Is the woman ready to enter the relational commitment to the child? Does she have the resources (bodily, financial, informational, and a community of caring people) to move to commit to the child? Has she accepted the moral claim of the child? The decision about abortion must be the mother's (if possible, in dialogue with important people in her life), because the child cannot continue to grow and develop without her—the woman and the fetus/child are one before they are two. In pregnancy the mother is *with* the child before she is *for* the child.

Until the woman has come to a decision on whether or not to accept the child within her body, we, the community, can only watch, wait, and support (with loving kindness). If the woman decides, at the birth of the child, that she cannot continue that relational commitment, she then makes her decision to place her child with others. We have learned from conversations with mothers who place their babies how difficult this is, for while the placing mother transfers day-to-day responsibility of the child, the child remains forever in her heart and mind. Both before and after the birth of the child (as a separate and unique person), it is the woman herself who must be the first decision-maker about the nature of the relational commitment. Even if the woman accepts the pregnancy, the birth, and/or the responsibility, the mothering commitment to the child takes time, varying with the circumstances of each woman.

Brenda Watson shows the challenge of making the relational commitment, of moving to take on the mothering relation, even if she does not refuse the pregnancy. Brenda Watson helps us to think about what it means to be ready to be a mother.

Brenda Watson. How could it happen so fast?

Brenda and Tom live in a new city development, the houses spaced inches apart. Two large dogs meet me at the door. Brenda is twenty-six. She has always thought she would have a child sooner or later. "We have been married five years this December and we decided that we have our house, have our dogs, have our vehicles, so it is more or less time. Actually I wanted to wait another year, but I will be twenty-seven next week and if we want two children, I'd better get started. Tom really did not want to wait, so I agreed to have the IUD taken out with the hope that it would take a few months to get pregnant.

"But two weeks later I never got my period and I was shocked. I was shocked and I cried. Tom laughed because he was so happy, ecstatic. Just like a little kid. He has wanted children for so long. I said, 'No, Tom, this can't happen that fast, no way.' But of course, I was. The first reaction was upset. I thought, 'How could it happen so fast, here I am going to be a mom and I don't want to be a mom just like that.' Thank God it takes five or six months before you really start to show. It was just shocking. I spent the whole summer being sick. Morning sickness. At work, with all the heavy lifting, I'd get cramps. And the sun. It was such a beautiful summer. I would go outside for five minutes, and I would be upstairs in the bathroom again. Or we would go camping and I'd be sick the whole time, from the time I got up until the time I went to bed. It was near the end of August I started to feel better. In a way you could say I was talked into getting pregnant. But I'm not sorry now, but at the time I was. 'Tom, how could you do this to me!' That kind of thing.

"At work, people drive me crazy. It's 'Mom this, and Mom that.' Just to get used to people coming up and wanting to touch your belly, like there must be a hundred staff in that store, and they are so thrilled to see a pregnant person, and they come up and want to feel your baby kicking. It really embarrasses me. But what do you say? In a lot of ways the baby comes first for other people. They say, Brenda, you shouldn't be doing that.' 'Your hands shouldn't be over your head, you shouldn't lift that.' 'Yes dear,' I say, mocking them. 'Yes, I won't do that anymore, I'm sorry, I was a bad girl,' and then I would turn around and do it.

"And I've noticed that you go into a crowded place, and a lot of people look at you and smile. Whereas before you could just walk in. When you go to a place, like Saturday night we went for a drink in a lounge, and I find that people really make you feel uneasy, like you are doing something just terrible, and you are only drinking orange juice. Like, 'come on!'

"I want to go back to work. I get so bored if I have two days off in a row. I like to get out and do something. I don't like to be stuck at home. But maybe with a child you would be doing things. We have a lady next door who will babysit. I'll start going back in the evenings and Tom will babysit. But like he says, 'I don't want to sit in the house every Saturday and babysit.' It is the same for me, I don't want to feel that I have to do everything with the baby. I want to have my own life too. If I want to go out with the girls, I should be able to.

"I am going to bottlefeed. That was a major fight. Tom believes in mother's milk. And me, just being the type of person I am, I just have an aversion to it. Even if I see someone else nursing it kind of gives me the creepy-crawlies. It is a natural thing, and I know it is good for the child, and I've heard all the good points about it. But it is just not for me. It's good old formula. Thank goodness they have invented those things.

"Our best friends have a three-month-old boy, and like I have yet to pick it up or anything like that. I am not the type that wants to cuddle or hold it, but they say it is different when it is your own. We will wait and see.

"I would rather have a boy, I don't think I want a girl, mainly because Tom would be too strict with her. I am sure if we had a little girl and she was out playing for two hours, and he didn't see her, it would be like twenty questions. 'Where were you?' 'What house were you in?' 'Who were you playing with?' He wouldn't do that with boys. He does it with me too. Like, we will go into a restaurant, and I will ask for something, and he will say, 'No, she doesn't want that, she is pregnant, she is having this.' I get this stunned look on my face and when the waitress leaves, I say,

'Tom, do you realize what you did?'

'No.'

'Tom, I asked for coffee and they are bringing me milk. I don't want milk.' He feels embarrassed, but I don't think he would notice he was doing it to a girl. Anyway, I think it is going to be a boy. We would be happy either way, but I have always felt that we are going to have boys.

"I find it, my body, really hard to accept. You understand that this is a baby growing inside you, and you have to get bigger, and you see your body growing different, and there are deposits of fat and stuff. It disgusts me. So far it is hard, it's firm, but you know that it will be jelly-like later on. It is hard to accept. I step on the scales, and I say, 'I weigh that much?' I believe that you can have a child and you can go back down to 115 pounds afterwards, there is no reason why you shouldn't. I feel that I should be the way I was before.

"We saw a film about natural childbirth and cesarean section at the prenatal class. I kept my eyes closed. 'Just let me know when it is over.' Tom was really impressed. Now he wants me to have a cesarean. He says it is more humane, like he doesn't like to see a woman suffer. He figures it would be less pain. I think it would be harder on your whole body, with getting used to the baby and not feeling as well as you could. I don't want it, but I don't think I will have any choice in the matter. Whatever is going to be is going to be."

Later, at the hospital, everything is happening very fast. The doctor comes in and puts her feet in the stirrups. The doctor says that on the next contraction the baby will be born. He cuts an episiotomy, and the baby slips out. The baby responds quickly and cries.

"It's a girl!" says the doctor.

"No!"

"I am going to put the baby on your stomach."

"No, please don't."

The doctor then holds the baby until the cord is clamped, which is almost right away, and gives the baby to the midwife, who wraps it and puts it under the lights in the bassinet. From the end of the room, the midwife involves herself with records and procedures. The doctors repair the episiotomy and the obstetrician again asks Brenda if she wants to hold her baby.

"No." She turns away.

We hear Brenda's struggle. We hear her difficulty in responding to her child. We hear her resistance to her changing body and changing lifestyle. We hear her concern about the reality of being a woman in the present culture. Even the reality of having a girl child is displayed in stark honesty. We hear the expectations of the community that she do certain things and not others and that she accept decisions made by someone else. We hear the fear of the never-ending, day-to-day childcare tasks. We hear the pressure to do something about mothering before it is too late. We hear attitudes about cesarean births, breastfeeding, and control. We hear the expectations of doctors and nurses, and we feel our own. We hear the truth in Brenda's worries. We are glad she speaks her truth so vividly.

But there is more to her story. Brenda is not alone. The doctors and nurses are there. Tom is there. I am there. In masks covering our noses and mouths, we stand and admire the baby. She is beautiful. I want to hold her, and suggest to Tom that he might. Though neither one of us does, we, as a community, are part of the picture. We share her story. We all do.

The following anecdote arrived by electronic mail some months ago. It points to the responsibility of both the mother and the community and to the nature of knowledge and freedom in relation to the child. It speaks of the moral commitment learned in mothering. It is the story of a man vacationing with his teenage daughter in another country. They are staying near a beach.

Homeless Girl. Who is responsible?

"One night all the locals in the bar were having a good laugh about the fact that a homeless girl who helped around the neighborhood had just given birth. The joke was, first, they hadn't noticed she was pregnant, and second, there were several possible candidates for the father's slot.

"My daughter went off to bed, but soon came back and said she'd found the baby lying in the sand out by the back porch, crying. The mother was lying on a bench, some distance away, doing nothing. I suggested we call a doctor. 'He's been,' someone said. 'He asked who was responsible. There wasn't anybody. So he wouldn't get involved.'

"I went out to look. The baby boy was wrapped in an old towel. It was crawling with ants and caked with blood. The afterbirth was still attached. My daughter and I did what we could to clean it up, and I cut the cord. We arranged transport into the nearest town and took the mother and baby to the hospital. The nurse asked if the girl had fed it. I told her the girl had said nothing and done nothing, so far as I could tell. Nurse, mother, and child disappeared into the surgery. We waited. After some time the nurse came out again.

'She's fine,' she says.

'You can go,' says the nurse, 'There's nothing more for you to do here.'

'My daughter thought I was a hero. All I could think of was how utterly stupidly I had blundered into a situation of enormous delicacy, and totally failed to see what was going on. The villagers had done nothing to help; nor had the doctor. Why? Because, in that situation, in that society, everyone knew that the choice lay with the mother. If she chose to feed the child, then she accepted responsibility for it.

"But she was allowed the freedom of choice. The others, doctor included, waited on her to make her choice. I hadn't done so. There is a point when a new life is accepted as an entity with rights within society. For some, it is the moment of birth, for others, somewhere between conception and birth. In the situation described above, the baby would have been endowed with rights only after the mother had elected to be responsible for it. Until and unless that happened, the baby's birth was not complete.

"I could have taken over that responsibility when it was clear that she could not accept it. There was that moment when I could have said so." (Barry Russell, personal communication, December 21, 1994)

One could ask many questions about this anecdote: How could the mother not feed, or at least hold, her child? If she accepted the pregnancy, how can she not accept the child? How can she not feed her child? She must not let the child die! We hear judgment in our tone. Or one could ask: Where is the father of the child? Did the young woman accept intercourse? Was she raped? Did she know how she got pregnant? Did she know what to do about it? Did she know where to go for help? If she does accept the child, who will help her with the care? Where is her own mother? Where are her friends? Where is the community support? Why is she homeless? Why do we call this mother a girl? How old is she? If there is any sense that something is wrong here, who is responsible? Now our voices are softer and more focused on understanding her situation.

There is freedom for all of us. There is freedom about whether or not we will enter the relational commitment of accepting the child. Brenda's honesty about how difficult a process it is to become a mother rings true for many women as they move to motherhood. The Homeless Girl shows us another truth—that the first choice, about taking on mothering, belongs to the mother. In her culture the birth of the child is not complete until someone takes up the relational claim of the child. Both Brenda Watson and the Homeless Girl remind us that in order for the mother to make the commitment to the child there must be support—there has to be a supportive community for mothering to happen. Mothers and fathers, women and men, we are all involved. In accepting the new life of a particular child, in the above descriptions, the woman has first choice. If she accepts the responsibility of the child, she gives the child birth into the communal life, not only with her body but also with her mind. The mother makes a decision about whether or not she can nurture that child. If she says yes, she needs support. And if she says no, for whatever reason, someone else in the community can take up the claim of responsiveness. Somebody must, or the child will die. It is our freedom. It is our choice.

The other side of the notion of freedom of choice is thinking that having children is a purely personal and private act and therefore a private responsibility: "Why should I pay for the education of other people's children?" or "Why should the work world provide parental leave or flexible work hours to accommodate family responsibilities?" When we think of children in this way, we see them as possessions or private acquisitions, and we forget what is learned from caring for children in intimate and daily ways.

What we forget, I suggest, is that our commitment to children, not as possessions but as relationships, is a moral commitment we all need to share. It is the commitment reflected in the turn from a focus on *me* to a focus on *us*. When public attention focuses on individual rights alone, on efficiency as the bottom line, and on individual financial wealth as the ultimate goal, there is little room for attention to the needs of others, especially children.

What gets lost, claims Bauman (1993), with this kind of individualistic thinking, is ourselves, our moral selves. "Losing the chance of morality is also losing the chance of the self. . . . Awakening to being for the Other is the awakening of the self, which is the *birth* of the self. There is no other awakening, no other way of finding out myself as the *unique* I, the one and only I, the I different from all others, the *irreplaceable* I, not a specimen of a category" (Bauman 1993: 77). The moral impulse, as awakening to being for the other person, is therefore two-headed: the move to being for the other person begets the potentiality of the self, that is, the moral self. With attention to our moral selves, we have the choice of what we want for a good life. One way of awakening to being for the child, as particular Other, is found in the woman's experience of pregnancy, birth, and nurturance. But this awakening is not confined to her alone, for we all can respond to the face of the child, the big eyes, the soft trusting body, the curled and bowed limbs—the actual living baby one takes into one's arms. It may be first experienced in the touch of the baby within the woman's body as she moves from the feeling of *this is my body* to *this is my baby*. Yet it may even begin before conception, as both birth and adoptive mother (and father) move toward thoughts of the child. The natural grounding of the moral impulse, the awakening to the Other, is hard to locate—perhaps it is already in each of us, a remnant held in our bodies, a memory of our first home, the body of our mother.

Could it be, then, that the mother-child relation is the foundational grounding of the moral impulse? Could it be the foundational experience of the turn toward the Other—to be with and for the Other? Zygmunt Bauman (1993), referring to the work of Emmanuel Levinas (1979), Søren Kierkegaard (1983), and others, places the primordial relationship that triggers the moral impulse in the erotic relationship, the caress. "The moral stance, as represented in Levinas's ethical teaching, is a metaphor of erotic love: simultaneously generalizing and particularizing, a mother-category and a specific case of love at the same time" (1993: 92). Instead of the erotic relationship, I suggest that the mother-child relation is our primordial experience of connection and commitment. While some may think that the woman-child relation, and specifically the woman-fetus relation, is fragile and unpredictable, R. Sarah believes that "it *is* powerful and trustworthy, and is the foundation of the strongest bond between human beings, and the *basis for all others*" (1987: 69. Emphasis added). Pregnancy, childbirth, and care of the child are important ways in which the moral move toward other persons is experienced.

If we take the pregnancy experience for what it is, with the fetus a part of the woman (not a separate entity), we cannot speak about women as vessels, containers, or maternal environments. Nor can we speak about fetuses as products of conception or separate patients—distinct and separate from their mother as patient. Nor can we speak of children as possessions, as property, as one's *own* child. If we take the pregnancy experience for what it is—women and their fetuses bound together, enmeshed in a social world (Rothman 1989)—and not just as a physical relationship (so easily managed by a technological attitude), we may be able to begin to understand the importance of freedom for women as they move into, or out of, pregnancy.

If we take the mothering experience for what it is—women and their children enmeshed in a social world and not just two separate people (so easily managed by a judgmental attitude)—we may be able to understand why mothers need the support of others to respond to the relational claim of the child. The experience of the mother as a responsiveness to the Other, be it fetus, baby, child, adolescent, or adult, can teach us the good, the quality of our relations, as a moral impulse. Mother love, that powerful love that women feel for their children, is a love that is nurturant, attentive, and dependable. Yet this love is not just developed instinctively, but is shaped and framed by the society in which that mother and that child live.

It may seem that relational engagement or commitment is an insecure foundation for morality, but it also may be our only hope (Bauman 1993). With modernity and its scientific, technological agenda, we have come to believe that if we just had more scientific research and more objective information, we would be able to control life—there would be no surprises, no diseases that cannot be prevented or cured, no behavior that cannot be predicted, and no situations that cannot be controlled. We think that increasing attention to abstract, generalizable knowledge will give us truth and certainty. We have come to fear that depending on our relational nature leaves us open to complete and unreliable relativism, because it seems to be too personal, too subjective, or even too emotional. But relational engagement is not relative; rather, it is bound by the relationship itself, the relationship between two or more embodied, concrete persons (Gadow 1994). In actual relationships the particularities of the context and the person are considered. Mothering, our primary experience of relational engagement, is dependable precisely because it is personal, because it touches the center of our being and focuses on the needs of the child as well as the mother. Mothers know this love and commitment. Fathers know it too. So do grandmothers and grandfathers, uncles and aunts.

We have learned from the experience of adoption that mothering love and commitment do not come only for women who give birth through their bodies. Becoming mother is a mindful (mind-expanding) as well as bodily experience. Love and commitment are learned in taking the *responsibility* for the child as one's own (not in taking the child as one's own). When we say that the moral move to the Other has its natural grounding in the experience of mothering, we refer to both its biological and its sociocultural grounding—where the biological and the sociocultural are indeterminate. We are free to choose how we value mothering and how we value our commitment to children and to others. We have a moral choice.

Quickening

Not everyone is a mother. Yet everyone is or has been mothered—by one's birth mother or adoptive mother, or by someone else. Everyone needs to be mothered, because everyone needs to be nurtured. Everyone needs support, connection, and engagement with and from others. "People are social beings by design not by choice," says the pediatrician Raymond Duff (1987: 244), who proposes that ethical commitments (especially in health-care) need close-up perspectives (attention to feelings, context, "habits of the heart") as well as the more distant perspectives of abstract ethical principles (beneficence, non-maleficence, autonomy, and distributive justice). The design of the social nature of human life is first recognized in quickening, where the mother says, "I am going to have a child. I feel the new life within." It is now "me and the baby."

Pregnant women describe quickening in a number of ways. Rachel O'Donnell, a teen mother, says it is "a gurgle, like water coming to a boil, with bubbles coming up." Quickening moves Rachel toward thinking about her baby and her commitment to her baby. We could also say that Jane Gibson is quickened by the look that Lisa gives her immediately after she is born, a look that makes Jane say, "It's just overwhelming. You can't turn her down." In describing the dread she feels when she anticipates the time when her adopted children want to go to their birth mothers, Jennifer Black says, "And if they decided to do that, well—I'll drive them." We hear, again, the mother's sense of being quickened to do what is best for her child. Experiences of quickening are not always easy. In fact, they may feel like bondage: "That flutter was good for an hour of miserable tears . . . this baby I had prayed for and longed for would not be joining my life, it seemed, but overtaking it all together . . . I had begun to disappear," says Rosemary Bray (1994: 143). The woman's world has changed, she has begun to see everything differently. It is not a smooth change. The moral self, as a relational self, is not the self-sufficient self that is pictured in much of liberal ethical theory (Held 1990). The relational self caught by the claim, the needs, of the Other is disturbing, and makes one question oneself and one's place.

Living with a child on your mind turns your attention to the Other, the child, and in that turning there comes a new attention to the self, with the self-questioning of "What should I do now?" "What is the right thing to do?" The woman as mother, the person most intimately responsive to the child, is guided by "the moral claim of the baby" (SmithBattle 1994: 160). Yet we know that morality is not confined to the mothers alone: other experiences of quickening are found in the erotic or the caress (Bauman 1993), severe illness (Duff 1993), or near death experiences (Kabat-Zinn 1994) that have affected people in profound ways and induced them to turn to the Other. Curtis Gillespie, a new father, tells how the birth and first six months of his daughter Jessica's life have changed not only his life, but also how he thinks about who he is. "I used to be a normal egocentric down-to-earth guy. Now . . . I am less certain of the order of things, less certain that the world revolves around my concerns. What really matters are things I only play a small part in. I have accepted that I'm not the centre of things, even within my own world. I know my place" (Gillespie 1996: 3). The place of moral commitment is an interdependent place, for it is through relations with others that we come to ourselves. "I am I by virtue of my act of affirming you; you are you by virtue of your act of affirming me. You are you, not *before* you perform the act of affirming me, but precisely *in the act*. . . . Persons experience their differentiation precisely in the act of meeting and touching, the act that makes them persons" (Bruteau 1978: 4, 5). It is through the meeting of actual flesh-and-blood human beings (like Jessica) with whom there are feelings and emotions, through relations with particular others, not generalized or *all* others, that the self is awakened (Held 1990).

Based on the philosophy of Emmanuel Levinas (1979), Wilfried Lippitz describes the moral claim of the Other as an obligation "to discover *myself* as an *I* in my responsibility for the Other, to step out of the maelstrom of my own self-referential, economic existence" (1990: 59). The ethical relationship arises only because the Other elicits a response from me. In an ethic of responsibility as described here, the Other is unique, "in need of everything that is necessary for a human life. By addressing myself to another I practice this responsibility, be it reluctantly or not. A total refusal of it would express itself through murder. Total acceptance would coincide with perfect love" (Peperzak 1989: 17). It is through relationship that we discover more about who we are and what we are capable of: "The Other enables me to do more than I can do," says Lippitz (1990: 55). Zygmunt Bauman agrees. "Moral behaviour is triggered off by the mere presence of the Other as a *face*: that is, an authority *without* force . . . it is precisely that weakness of the Other that lays bare my strength, my ability to act, as responsibility" (Bauman 1993: 124). Relationships make it possible (not just necessary) to be moral.

The philosopher Hans Jonas proposed in 1966 that an ethic of responsibility is motivated by the "basic, original, and natural" experience of parental responsibility (Bernstein 1995: 16). The paradigm of parental responsibility as the motivation to moral responsibility that Jonas and Bernstein (1995) describe is a "non-reciprocal relation of caring," which, Bernstein warns, could lead to detrimental paternalistic (or maternalistic) authority. I agree with Bernstein in supporting the need for "another dimension of responsibility—the *mutual, reciprocal* responsibility to my fellow human beings" (1995: 17). The experience of quickening that is found in mothering is just that: quickening is relational, reciprocal, and mutual. Not only does the mother feel the physical movement within; she also responds to that movement in a concrete way—conversing, playing, and telling the baby to "share." The reciprocal nature of quickening—the mother's being *with* before she can be *for* the other—differs from both Jonas's and Bauman's development of an ethic of responsibility. Quickening during pregnancy begins the conversational turn-taking that has been observed between mothers and infants from the moment of birth (Hermans and Kempen 1993). The reciprocity, the mutuality of quickening begins the moral relation.

Quickening elicits an immediate response, before one has a chance to think about it. Impulse and the action are one. In quickening the knowing-what-to-do has no theoretical quality—it is entirely practical, immediate, and compelling (Sacks 1984). It is an awakening to the reality of another being. It is said that quickening is also "associated with pilgrims who go to sacred places to 'quicken' the divinity within themselves, to experience spiritual awakening or receive a blessing or become healed" (Bolen 1994: 28). As such, quickening can be seen as an awakening to the new life–in pregnancy and in personal life.

Quickening has to do with connections, with relationships that are mutually (that is, for both persons in the relationship—mother and child, father and child, self and Other) empathic and enlivening. Quickening, as a moral impulse, demonstrates the need for understanding the experience of the body as well as the ability of mind. It shows the need to understand the experience of living in the world as well as knowledge about the world (Gadow 1979; Bergum 1994b). It displays the need for particular knowledge (individual, close-up knowledge) as well as generalizable knowledge (universal, distinct knowledge) (Duff 1987; Gadow 1992). Quickening has to do with touching and hearing as well as thinking and seeing, with nurturance as well as beneficence. It has to do with growth, change, and healing. There is a need to revive the word quickening to common usage—both in valuing woman's personal knowledge of the child moving within and as a way to think about our moral lives.

Miller and Stiver (1991) articulate five components of the enlivening (or quickening) that happens with mutual connections between people. They refer to the therapeutic relationship, but I propose that these components are possible in all relationships: "an increased zest or well-being that comes with feeling connected to others; the motivation and ability to act right in the relationship as well as beyond it; an increased knowledge about oneself and the other person(s), an increased sense of self worth; and a desire for connection beyond this particular one (Miller and Stiver 1991: 2). Understanding and valuing the experience of mothering and the connection that mothers have with children may assist us to realize that quickening—that recognition (being-with) and commitment (being-for) the other person cannot be separated. Sally Gadow says, "In mothering there is *union* of being-with and being-for (personal communication, June 14, 1996). The mystery of each new beginning and quickening needs, perhaps, infinite darkness and silence (as in the womb) for new life to be created (Sacks 1984).

David Smith (1984) asserts that, in our relational commitment to children, we lose control of ourselves and become aware that there is more to life than what we previously knew. Perhaps though, we actually gain control of ourselves, attending to our needs and responsibilities in new ways. Smith is right in describing these complex relations as mysterious; they are not, however, mysterious in the sense that we cannot know them, but because of life's complexities. This losing and gaining control of ourselves is a positive move, a move toward the Other and toward the self. The aim is to understand the child and ourselves more completely. The move toward understanding the child or the mother does not refer to knowledge of developmental tasks of the child or the mother (although this is useful information); rather, it means learning what the child demands of us—or what it means to be *with* and *for* the child, to foster the potential of the child. Understanding the nature of our relational commitments fragments our thinking, according to Katherine Lang, by forcing us to ask ourselves questions about who we are and what is important in life.

THE MOTHER STORY

The story is a form of knowledge. Some people say the story is all we have to fight off sickness and death (Silko 1977). The story is healing for both the teller and the listener. A story tells about a journey, about "once upon a time," about "what happened," and "then what happened," and on and on. Through mothering stories as developed in this book, we can share the varied journeys that women take into motherhood. We can be fellow travellers. We can see that there is more than one way to mother. There is more than one way to become and be a mother. We see that mothering is a personal journey, a personal narrative, with no script to be learned ahead of time. One mother's story is no better or more legitimate than any other mother's story. With stories the question of legitimacy is itself illegitimate: each mother's story is self-legitimizing (Parry and Doan 1994).

The mother story is not a hero story, not a battle with its one plot with a beginning, middle, and end. Rather, the mother story is more like what Ursula Le Guin (1989b) calls the carrier bag story. The mother story carries many plots, with many beginnings, middles, and endings (Le Guin says that in narrative conceived as a carrier bag (belly, box, house, medicine bundle), story, conflict, stress, and struggle are seen as necessary elements of a whole and are not characterized as conflict or as harmony, since the purpose is neither resolution nor stasis, but continuing process (1989b: 169). In the mother story, there are no sticks, spears, and swords that bash, thrust, rape, and kill; rather, there are gatherings, sortings, and winnowings—activities that are repeated over and over. The blood and pain of the mother story do not stem from inflicting wounds but from the ongoing rhythm of life and death, and the possibility of new life. The mother story as a container, like a carrier bag, holds meanings, relationships, fears, and joys, during intense periods in women's lives. The mother story, like all life journeys, is continuous. The mother story is generational. It never ends. When one is on the mothering journey, it often seems that one just has to get over the next hill to get home free. Yet in real life, instead of finding the finish line, one finds another starting line.

Mothering, as life, is a journey that blurs the distinction between separate, autonomous individuals—mothers and children. The vision of separate, autonomous individuals is a result of the relatively recent emphasis on abstract, universal, scientific knowledge (Burt 1979). Instead of the technological separation of mother and child, even before birth, the vision of mothering as a journey shows a concrete intimacy, in which mother and child journey together, giving and taking, pausing and moving ahead, like dance partners sensitive to the movement and rhythm of each other. The mothering relation, as experienced, blurs the boundaries between mother and child, tending to make them diffuse and flexible, holding close and letting go, being one and then being two. The mothering story is the relational story by its very nature.

Ursula Le Guin (1989a) tells women to offer their experience as their truth, and when women offer their experience as truth, as human truth, all the maps change. There are new mountains and valleys, new crossroads and highways, new potholes and broken pavement. There are new possibilities and visions. If women don't tell their truth, who will? Who will speak for the children and for the mothers? The sharing of mothers' stories may be the most accessible way we have to understand our commitments to our children and to each other. Helen Klodawsky (1994), in the video *Motherland: Tales of Wonder*, reminds us that the only thing that seems certain is that outside perspectives are dangerous and blueprints do not exist. Perhaps the true stories of mothers spoken in public are the only genuine guide.

Yet, stories of mothering are not merely the documenting of personal experiences, but are a form of practical knowledge from which mothers, healthcare professionals, and others can learn. Engaging in conversations about women's experiences (narratives) gives us a chance to create new narratives that will lead to a stronger sense of rightness about what we should be doing with and for mothers and children. All stories, once spoken and shared, reveal intersubjectivity, that is, show how we are the same and how we are different—knowledge that will increase our ability to understand our human condition anew. This kind of knowledge, narrative knowledge, does not lead to certainty, the truth, but it does lead to understanding, a truth that is approximate, not absolute (Capra and Steindl-Rast 1991).

Listening to another's story and telling our own give us opportunities to respond to each other, and to understand ourselves. When stories are shared, one might ask questions like, "What really happened here?" "What sense do I make of it?" "Should I have acted this way?" "What would you have done?" As one gives an account of what happened, that is, tells the story, one becomes accountable and gives reasons why this action is good and what one would do another time. Giving an account opens us to the dark side of mothering—the pain, the fear, the continuous commitment—as well as the pleasures and loves. When stories are shared, the dark pictures are not banished or hidden, but are faced directly. Ways and means are found to navigate through them. As they are shared, stories give meaning to our lives and our relationships, and through storytelling we gain reflectiveness, thoughtfulness, and tact.

Many of the women who shared their own stories of mothering expressed gratitude for being invited to tell of their experiences. Through sharing what they were going through, they were able to reflect on their own experience and return to it in an invigorated fashion. Hannah Eldridge, a placing mother, comments, "Talking about my experience was actually good for me—talking about everything helped me to sort out my feelings." Celine Merrill, a teen mother, found that being able to talk about her experience in a nonjudgmental environment was beneficial: "Other people just think, 'Well, you're doing that wrong,' and 'you should be doing this,' but you just sit there and you listen, you're not trying to tell me what to do. It's really good." Karin Perry, an adopting mother, says, "The whole process of thinking about it and writing about it and telling people about it over and over again as you do in talking to social workers and even in talking to you, Vangie, just kind of opens you up. It makes you realize what you think about things and kind of gets some of the kinks out." Sharing one's story assists one to steer around the kinks and bends in the road, to maneuver around the potholes, and to manipulate the broken pavement.

This book contains the stories of women who mother (birth, placing, adopting, and teen mothers), who have a child on their mind. As one is drawn into the relational commitment to the child, instead of losing oneself in that commitment, one gains oneself anew. The self is enlarged. This relational view of the world, a grounding for morality through its pull toward an Other, makes possible the strengthening of the Self. It is a view of our human connection that is learned, perhaps most profoundly, at the mother's knee. To have one's mind full of thoughts of the child—while it may at times fragment thinking—pays respect to the child and the child's needs, and can enrich mothers' (indeed, parents') lives. Having a child on one's mind causes one to think of the nature of the world as a community for children.

NOTE

This chapter incorporates sections of two previous publications: Abortion revisited: Toward an understanding of the nature of the woman-fetus relationship. *Phenomenology & Pedagogy*, 8: 3, 14–21, 1990; and The first breath, in J. Ross & V. Bergum (Eds.), *Through the Looking Glass: Children and Health Promotion* (pp. 11–17). Ottawa: CPHA, 1990. Used with permission.

Appendix: The Research Process

Various studies have been completed during the research program about mothering. Women were interviewed through conversations about various aspects of their experience. The names of all women were changed to protect anonymity.

Nine women were in conversation about their experience of *childbirth pain* in January and February 1983: Diane Lyttle, Ellie Robertson, Flo Hammer, Helen Crozier, Iris Cummings, Laura Brown, Noa Alexander, Victoria LeClair, and Xavier Marshal.

Seven women were in conversation about their experience with the *fetal monitor* in December 1984: Melissa Spring, Natasha Scott, Opal Rawls, Una Todd, Wendy Skinner, and Yvonne Mark.

A major study (a doctoral dissertation) took place from 1984 to 1986 exploring the experiences of *pregnancy and childbirth*. The women were Anna Gurley, Brenda Watson, Christine Martin, Jane Gibson, Katherine Lang, and Susan McLaren. Other women quoted here include Gail Lehman and Paula Peters. A total of forty-five in-depth conversations took place within this study.

Conversations with women describing their experience of the *fetus during pregnancy* took place during 1990–1991. One woman was interviewed shortly after a miscarriage in early pregnancy. There were ten women in this study. Glenda Richards, Sylvie Foster, and Nancy Thompson are cited in this work.

Conversations with women for the adoption study occurred between 1991 and 1993. Adopting women (ages thirty-five to forty-six years) include Nel Henry, Joan Bell, Jennifer Black, Karin Perry, Lois Reynolds, Gwen Reid, Barbara Campbell, Connie Hancock, Allison Decker, and Charlotte Elias. Placing women (ages fifteen to twenty-four years) include Lorrie Newton, Mary Sebastian, Terry Lee, Sally Corbett, Cathy Bishop, Hannah Eldridge, Jesse Abbott, Sandy Moss, Rosie Smith and Pauline Earl. Young single women (ages fifteen to eighteen) include Jasmine

Jonson, Holly Radcliff, Rachel O'Donnell, Celine Merrill, Ruth-Ann Stapleton, and Jesse Miller that chose to keep their children to raise. The participants in this research are women recruited through two agencies: a school for single teen mothers and an adoption agency that supports open adoptions. In open adoption the birth mother selects the adoptive parents and has various degrees of contact with them after the adoption of the child.

This program of research was carried out with approval from the Research Ethics Committee (Faculty of Nursing, University of Alberta). The conversations were transcribed with identifying information removed. The tapes are kept under secured conditions. The transcriptions, classified by code name and number according to date of conversation, are kept in binders and on computer discs. Other information about the research protocol can be obtained by writing the author at The Bioethics Centre, University of Alberta, 222 ANR, 8220–114th Street, Edmonton, Alberta, Canada, T6G2J3 or by e-mail at vbergum @ gpu.srv.ualberta.ca.

Bibliography

Anderson, Gene C., Elizabeth A. Marks, & Vivian Wahlberg. (1986). Kangaroo care for premature infants. *American Journal of Nursing*, 86: 7, 807–809.

Arendt, Hannah. (1961). *The crisis in education: Between past and future*. New York: Viking.

Ashford, Janet Isaacs. (Ed.). (1984). *Birth stories: The experience remembered*. Trumansburg, N.Y.: The Crossing Press.

Atwood, Margaret. (1985). *The handmaid's tale*. Toronto: McClelland & Stewart.

Bachelard, Gaston. (1969). *The poetics of space*. Boston: Beacon.

Baier, Annette. (1987). The need for more than justice. In Marsha Hanen & Kai Nelson (Eds.), *Science, Morality and Feminist Theory*. Calgary: University of Calgary Press.

Barber, Virginia, & Merrill Maguire Skaggs. (1975). *The mother person*. New York: Bobbs-Merrill.

Barrett, William. (1987). *Death of the soul: From Descartes to the computer*. New York: Anchor Books.

Bauman, Zygmunt. (1993). *Postmodern ethics*. Oxford, U.K.: Blackwell Publishers.

Baumgarten, Kurt. (1981). The advantages and risks of feto-maternal monitoring. *Journal of Perinatal Medicine*, 9, 257–274.

Belenky, Mary F., Blythe M. Clinchy, Nancy R. Goldberger, & Jill M. Tarule. (1986). *Women's ways of knowing: The development of self, voice and mind*. New York: Basic Books.

Benjamin, Walter. (1969). The storyteller. In *Illuminations* (pp. 83–109). New York: Schocken.

Benner, Patricia. (Ed.). (1994). *Interpretive phenomenology: Embodiment, caring and ethics in health and illness*. Thousand Oaks, Calif.: Sage Publications.

Bergum, Vangie. (1989). *Woman to mother: A transformation.* Granby, Mass.: Bergin & Garvey.

Bergum, Vangie. (1994a). Commentary of Epistemology of Expectant Parenthood. *Western Journal of Nursing Research,* 16:6, 616–618.

Bergum, Vangie. (1994b). Knowledge for ethical care. *Nursing Ethics. An International Journal for Health Care Professionals,* 1:2, 72–79.

Bergum, Vangie. (In press). The experience of mothers in open adoption: A Canadian perspective. In Evi Constantinidou & Janette Davis (Eds.), *Adoption in a Cross-Cultural Perspective.* London: Berg Publishers Limited.

Bernstein, Richard. (1995). Rethinking responsibility. *The Hastings Center Report,* 25:7, 13–20.

Billington, Rachel. (1994). *The great umbilical: Mother, daughter, mother, the unbreakable bond.* London: Hutchinson.

Blanton, Terril L., & Jeanne Deschner. (1990). Biological mothers' grief: The postadoptive experience in open versus confidential adoption. *Child Welfare,* 69, 525–535.

Bolen, Jean Shinoda. (1994). *Crossing to Avalon.* New York: HarperCollins Publishers.

Bolker, Joan. (1994). A room of one's own is not enough. *Tikkun,* 7:6, 51–87.

Bollnow, Otto. (1987). *Crisis and new beginnings.* Pittsburgh: Duquesne University Press.

Bonica, John. (1975). The nature of pain in parturition. *Clinics in Obstetrics and Gynaecology,* 3:2, 499–517.

Bordo, Susan. (1993). *Unbearable weight: Feminism, western culture, and the body.* Los Angeles: University of California Press.

Braine, David, & Harry Lesser. (1988). *Ethics, technology and medicine.* Aldershot, U.K.: Avebury.

Brandt, Di. (1993). *Wild mother dancing: Maternal narrative in Canadian literature.* Winnipeg: University of Manitoba Press.

Brandt, Di. (1995). *Jerusalem, beloved.* Winnipeg: Turnstone Press.

Bray, Rosemary. (1994). First stirrings. In Patricia Foster (Ed.), *Minding the body: Women writers on body and soul* (pp. 139–145). New York: Doubleday.

Brownmiller, Susan. (1984). *Femininity.* New York: Fawcett Columbine.

Bruteau, Beatrice. (1978). Neo-feminism as communion consciousness. *Anima,* Fall: 3–5.

Buck, Pearl. (1931). *The good earth.* New York: Pocket Books.

Burch, Robert. (1984). *Towards a philosophical perspective.* Occasional Paper No. 27, Department of Secondary Education, University of Alberta.

Burt, Robert (1979). *Taking care of strangers: The rule of law in doctor-patient relations.* New York: The Free Press.

Butala, Sharon. (1994). *The perfection of the morning: An apprenticeship in nature.* Toronto: HarperCollins Publishers Ltd.

Buytendijk, Frederik Jacobus Johannes. (1961). *Pain.* London: Hutchinson and Company.

Cameron, Anne. (1981). *Daughters of copper woman.* Vancouver: Press Gang Publishers.

Capra, Fritjof, & David Steindl-Rast. (1991). *Belonging to the universe: Explorations on the frontiers of science and spirituality.* New York: HarperCollins Publishers.

Carter, Betty, & Monica McGoldrick. (Eds.). (1989). *The changing family life cycle: A framework for family therapy.* Boston: Allyn and Bacon.

Carter-Jessop, L. (1981). Promoting maternal attachment through prenatal intervention. *Maternal Child Nursing,* 6, 107–112.

Chapman, Cathy, Patricia Dorner, Kathy Silber, & Terry S. Winterberg. (1986). Meeting the needs of the adoption triangle through open adoption: The birthmother. *Child and Adolescent Social Work,* 3, 203–213.

Chernin, Kim. (1987). *Reinventing Eve: Modern woman in search of herself.* New York: Times Books.

Chesler, Phyllis. (1979). *With child: A diary of motherhood.* New York: Thomas Y. Crowell.

Chicago, Judy. (1985). *The birth project.* New York: Doubleday.

Chodorow, Nancy. (1978). *The reproduction mothering: Psychoanalysis and the sociology of gender.* Berkeley: University of California Press.

Colen, B. D. (1986). *Hard choices: Mixed blessings of modern medical technology.* New York: G. P. Putnam.

Connolly, Maureen. (1987). The experience of living with an absent child. *Phenomenology and Pedagogy,* 5, 157–172.

Davis-Floyd, Robbie. (1994). The technocratic body: American childbirth as cultural expression. *Social Science and Medicine,* 38:8, 1125–1140.

Dillon, Robin. (1992). Respect and care: Toward moral integration. *Canadian Journal of Philosophy,* 22:1, 105–132.

Downey, Geraldine, Roxanne C. Silver, & Camille B. Wortman. (1990). Reconsidering the attribution-adjustment relation following a major negative event: Coping with the loss of a child. *Journal of Personality and Social Psychology,* 59, 925–940.

Dowrick, Stephanie, & Sibyl Grundberg. (Eds.). (1980). *Why children?* New York: Harcourt Brace Jovanovich.

Duden, Barbara. (1993). *Disembodying woman: Perspectives on pregnancy and the unborn.* (Lee Hoinacki, Trans.). Cambridge, Mass.: Harvard University Press.

Duerk, Judith. (1989). *Circle of stones: Woman's journey to herself.* San Diego, Calif.: LuraMedia.

Duff, Kat. (1993). *The alchemy of illness.* New York: Pantheon Books.

Duff, Raymond. (1987). "Close-up" versus "distant" ethics: Deciding the care of infants with poor prognosis. *Seminars in Perinatology,* 11:3, 244–253.

Dunham, C., F. Myers, N. Barnden, A. McDougall, T. Kelly, with B. Aria. (1991). *Mamatoto: A celebration of birth.* London: Virago Press Ltd.

Edwards, Caternia, & Kay Stewart. (Eds.). (1994). *Eating apples: Knowing women's lives.* Edmonton: NuWest Press.

Engelmann, George Julius. (1884). *Labour among primitive peoples.* St. Louis, Mo.: J. H. Chambers.

Erdrich, Louise. (1995). *The blue jay's dance.* New York: HarperCollins Publishers.

Erikson, Erich. (1963). *Childhood and society.* New York: W. W. Norton.

Fallaci, Oriana. (1976). *Letter to a child never born.* New York: Washington Square Press.

Farber, Naomi B. (1991). The process of pregnancy resolution among adolescent mothers. *Adolescence,* 26:103, 697–716.

Field, Jeff. (1992). Psychological adjustment of relinquishing mothers before and after reunion with their children. *Australian and New Zealand Journal of Psychiatry*, 26, 232–241.

Field, Peggy A., & Patricia Marck. (Eds.). (1994). *Uncertain motherhood: Negotiating the risks of the childbearing years* (pp. 268–298). Thousand Oaks, Calif.: Sage Publications.

Fujita, Mikio. (1985). Modes of waiting. *Phenomenology and Pedagogy*, 3:2, 107–115.

Gadow, Sally. (1979). The dialectic of clinical judgement. In H. T. Englehardt (Ed.), *Clinical Judgement: A Critical Appraisal* (pp. 248–253). Dordrecht, Holland: K. Reidel.

Gadow, Sally. (1992). Existential ecology: The human/natural world. *Social Science and Medicine*, 35:4, 597–602.

Gadow, Sally. (1994). Whose body? Whose story? The question about narrative in women's health care. *Soundings*, 77:3–4, 295–307.

Gale, Gay, Linda Fanck, & Carolyn Lund. (1993). Skin-to-skin (kangaroo) holding of the intubated infant. *Neonatal Network*, 12:6, 49–57.

Gélis, Jacques. (1991). *History of childbirth: Fertility, pregnancy and birth in early modern Europe*. (R. Morris, Trans.). Boston: Northeastern University Press.

Gervais, Suzanne. (1993). *Expectations*. Ottawa: National Film Board. (Video).

Gillespie, Curtis. (1996). *The kid*. Commentary on CBC Radio Active, Canadian Broadcasting Corporation. January 9.

Gilligan, Carol. (1983). *In a different voice*. Cambridge: Mass.: Harvard University Press.

Gilligan, C., J. V. Ward, J. M. Taylor, & B. Bardige. (Eds.). (1988). *Mapping the moral domain*. Cambridge, Mass.: Harvard University Press.

Gleick, Elizabeth, et al. (1994, October 24). Babies who have babies. *People* magazine, Special Report, 38–56.

Glenn, Evelyn. (1994). Social constructions of mothering: A thematic overview. In E. N. Glenn. G. Chang, & L. R. Forcey (Eds.), *Mothering: Ideology, experience, and agency* (pp. 1–29). London: Routledge.

Glenn, Evelyn Nakano, Grace Chang, & Linda Rennie Forcey. (Eds.). (1994). *Mothering: Ideology, experience, and agency*. London: Routledge.

Goody, Esther, N. (1982). *Parenthood and social reproduction: Fostering and occupational roles in West Africa*. Cambridge, U.K.: Cambridge University Press.

Grahn, Judy. (1993). *Blood, bread and roses. How menstruation created the world*. Boston: Beacon Press.

Habermas, Jürgen. (1987). *Knowledge and human interests*. (J. Shapiro, Trans.). Cambridge, U.K.: Polity Press.

Harrison, Michelle. (1982). *A woman in residence*. New York: Random House.

Hayden, Joyce. (1995). Building a firm foundation for teen mothers. *Herizons. Women News & Feminist Views*, 9:2, 11.

Heart surgery performed in the womb. (1990, February 1). *The Edmonton Journal*. A5.

Heckler, Richard. (1984). *The anatomy of change*. Boulder, Colo.: Shambhala.

Heidegger, Martin. (1977). *The question concerning technology and other essays*. (W. Lovitt, Trans.). New York: Harper Torchbooks.

Held, Virginia. (1990). Feminist transformations of moral theory. *Philosophy and Phenomenological Research*, 1: Supplement, 321–344.

Held, Virginia. (1993). *Feminist morality: Transforming culture, society, and politics.* Chicago: University of Chicago Press.

Hermans, Hubert, & Harry Kempen. (1993). *The dialogical self: Meaning as movement.* San Diego: Academic Press, Inc.

Hipple, Lee, & Barb Haflich. (1993). Adoption's forgotten clients: Birth siblings. *Child and Adolescent Social Work Journal,* 10, 53–65.

Hoff, Gerard Alan, & Lawrence J. Schneiderman. (1985). Having babies at home: Is it safe? Is it ethical? *Hastings Center Report,* 15:6, 19–27.

Hogarth, Meg. (1995, June 19). MediaWatch (a newsletter).

Howe, David. (1990). The loss of a baby. *Midwife Health Visitor & Community Nurse,* 26:1 & 2, 25–26.

Hubbard, Ruth. (1984). Personal courage is not enough: Some hazards of childbearing in the 1980's. In R. Arditti, R. Duelli, & S. Minden (Eds.). *Test-tube women* (pp. 33–55). Boston: Pandora Press.

Hyde, Lewis. (1983). *The gift: Imagination and the erotic life of property.* New York: Vintage Books.

Israeloff, Roberta. (1982). *Coming to terms.* New York: Penguin.

Jonas, Hans. (1966). *The phenomenon of life: Toward a philosophical biology.* New York: Harper & Row.

Kabat-Zinn, Jon. (1994). What is my job on the planet with a capital j? In *Wherever you go there you are* (pp. 206–209). New York: Hyperion.

Kaplan, E. Ann. (1994). Look who's talking indeed: Fetal images in recent North American visual culture. In E. N. Glenn, G. Chang, & L. R. Forcey (Eds.), *Mothering: Ideology, experience, and agency* (pp. 121–137). London: Routledge.

Keating, John. (1994, March). Parents keep preemies warm and healthy. *Canadian Living.* 23.

Kelpin, Vangie. (1985). *Ear on the belly: A question of fetal monitors.* Occasional Paper. Department of Secondary Education, University of Alberta.

Kelpin, Vangie, & Angeline Martel. (1984). The language of obstetrics from the experience of birthing. *Women: Images, role-models* (pp. 150–158). Montreal: Canadian Research Institute for the Advancement of Women.

Kierkegaard, Søren. (1954/1983). *Fear and trembling.* (H. Hong & E. Hong, Trans.). Princeton, N.J.: Princeton University Press.

Kirk, H. David. (1984). *Shared fate: A theory and method of adoptive relationships.* (2nd ed.). Brentwood Bay, British Columbia: Ben-Simon Publications.

Kittay, Eva Feder. (1983). Womb envy: An explanatory concept. In Joyce Trebilcot (Ed.), *Mothering: Essays in feminist theory* (pp. 94–128). Totowa, N.J.: Rowman and Allanhead.

Kitzinger, Sheila. (1977). *Giving birth: The parents' emotions in childbirth.* New York: Schocken.

Kitzinger, Sheila. (1979). *Education and counselling for childbirth.* New York: Schocken.

Klaus, Marshall, & John Kennell. (1976). *Maternal-infant bonding.* St. Louis: C. V. Mosby.

Klodawsky, Helen. (1994). *Motherland: Tales of Wonder.* Ottawa: National Film Board of Canada. (Video).

Koepke, Jean, Jan Austin, Sharon Anglin, & Joanne Delesalle. (1991). Becoming parents: Feelings of adoptive mothers. *Pediatric nursing*, 17, 333–336.

Kohlberg, Lawrence. (1981). *The meaning and measurement of moral development*. Worcester, Mass.: Clark University Press.

Kristeva, Julia. (1986). Stabat Mater. In Toril Moi (Ed.), *The Kristeva Reader* (pp. 160–186). New York: Columbia University Press.

Kristeva, Julia. (1991). *Strangers to ourselves: European perspectives*. New York: Columbia University Press.

Lauderdale, J. L., & J. S. Boyle. (1994). Infant relinquishment through adoption. *Image. Journal of Nursing Scholarship*, 26, 213–217.

Lawrence, B. Joan. (1996, in press). A grandmother's reflection. In Susan James and Sandy Pullin (Eds.), *A midwife's guide to homebirth—Pregnancy, birth and postpartum*. Edmonton: With Woman Midwifery Care.

Le Guin, Ursula. (1989a). Bryn Mawr commencement address. In Ursula Le Guin, *Dancing at the edge of the world* (pp. 147–160). New York: Harper & Row.

Le Guin, Ursula. (1989b). Carrier bag theory of fiction. In Ursula Le Guin, *Dancing at the edge of the world* (pp. 165–170). New York: Harper & Row.

Leifer, Myra. (1977). Psychological changes accompanying pregnancy and motherhood. *Genetic Psychology Monographs*, 95, 55–96.

Lévesque, Andrée. (1990). Deviants anonymous: Single mothers at the hospital de la Misericorde in Montreal, 1929–1939. In Katherine Arnup, Andrée Lévesque, & Ruth Roach Pierson (Eds.), *Delivering motherhood: Maternal ideologies and practices in the 19th and 20th centuries* (pp. 108–125). London: Routledge.

Levesque-Lopman, Louise. (1983). Decision and experience: A phenomenological analysis of pregnancy and childbirth. *Human Studies*, 6, 247–277.

Levinas, Emmanuel. (1979). *Totality and infinity*. Boston: Martinus Nijhoff Publishers.

Lippitz, Wilfried. (1990). Ethics as limits of pedagogical reflection. *Phenomenology and Pedagogy*, 8: 49–60.

Lopez, Barry. (1995). Currents. *Utne Reader*, 70: 38–39.

Lozoff, B., G. Brittenham, M. Trause, J. Kennell, & M. Klaus. (1977). The mother-newborn relationship: Limits of adaptability. *The Journal of Pediatrics*, 91:1, 1–12.

McDermott, John. (1986). The stethoscope as talisman: Medical technology and loneliness. *AARN Newsletter*, 41:2, 21–24.

McDonald-Grandin, Merrilyn. (1983). *Will I ever be a mother?* Portland, Ore.: Celeste Books.

McLaughlin, Steven D., Susan E. Pearce, Diane L. Manninen, & Linda D. Winges. (1988). To parent or relinquish: Consequences for adolescent mothers. *Social Work*, 33, 320–324.

McRoberts, V. (1984, January 15). Miracle on 87 St. *The Edmonton Journal*. B9.

Mander, Rosemary. (1991a). Midwifery care of the grieving mother: How the decisions are made. *Midwifery*, 7, 133–142.

Mander, Rosemary. (1991b). Midwifery support of the mother relinquishing her baby for adoption: Midwives' perceptions. *Midwives Chronicle and Nursing Notes*, 104: 245, 275–285.

March, Karen. (1995). *The stranger who bore me: Adoptee-birth mother relationships.* Toronto: University of Toronto Press.

Marck, Patricia, Peggy A. Field, & Vangie Bergum. (1994). A search for understanding. In Peggy Ann Field & Patricia Marck (Eds.), *Uncertain motherhood: Negotiating the Risks of the Childbearing Years* (pp. 268–298). Thousand Oaks, Calif.: Sage Publications.

Mehl, Lewis E., Gail H. Peterson, Michael Whitt, & Warren E. Hawes. (1977). Outcomes of elective home births: A series of 1,146 cases. *The Journal of Reproductive Medicine, 19,* 281–290.

Meinhart, Noreen, & Margo McCaffery. (1983). *Pain: A nursing approach to assessment and analysis.* Norwalk, Conn.: Appleton-Century-Crofts.

Meltzer, David. (Ed.). (1981). *Birth as an anthology of ancient texts, songs, prayers, and stories.* San Francisco: North Point.

Melzack, Ronald, Paul Taenzer, Parle Feldman, & Robert Kinch. (1980). Labour is still painful after prepared childbirth training. *Canadian Medical Association Journal, 4:125,* 357–363.

Mercer, Ramona. (1981). A theoretical framework for studying factors that impact on the maternal role. *Nursing Research, 30,* 73–77.

Mercer, Ramona. (1995). *Becoming a mother. Research on maternal identity from Rubin to the present.* New York: Springer Publishing Company.

Mercer, Ramona, S. Ferketich, K. May, J. DeJoseph, & D. Sollid. (1988). Further exploration of maternal and paternal fetal attachment. *Research in Nursing and Health, 11,* 83–95.

Merleau-Ponty, Maurice. (1962). *Phenomenology of perception.* (C. Smith, Trans.). London: Routledge & Kegan Paul.

Miller, Jean Baker. (1986). *Toward a new psychology of women.* (2nd ed.). Boston: Beacon.

Miller, Jean Baker, & Irene P. Stiver. (1991). *A relational reframing of therapy.* Wellesley, Mass.: The Stone Center, Wellesley College.

Modell, Judith S. (1994). *Kinship with strangers: Adoption and interpretations of kinship in American culture.* Berkeley: University of California Press.

Moore, Thomas. (1992). *Care of the soul: A guide for cultivating depth and sacredness in everyday life.* New York: HarperCollins Publishers.

Morgan, Robin. (1984). *The anatomy of freedom: Feminism, physics and global politics.* New York: Anchor Books/Doubleday.

Morris, William. (Ed.). (1975). *The American heritage dictionary of the English language.* Boston: Houghton Mifflin Company.

Morrison, Toni. (1988). *Beloved.* New York: Knopf.

Mutén, Burleigh. (1994). *Return of the great goddess.* Boston: Shambhala.

Nathanielsz, Peter. (1992). *Life before birth and a time to be born.* Ithaca, N.Y.: Promethean Press.

Nelson, Fiona. (1995). Musings on motherhood: Three short essays. Unpublished manuscript. University of Alberta.

Neumann, Erich. (1955). *The great mother: An analysis of the archetype.* Princeton, N.J.: Princeton University Press.

Neumann, Erich. (1990). *The child.* (Ralph Manheim, Trans.) Boston: Shambhala.

Newton, Niles. (1955). *Maternal emotions.* New York: Paul B. Hoeber, Inc.

Northrup, Christiane. (1994). *Women's bodies, women's wisdom: Creating physical and emotional health and healing*. New York: Bantam Books.

Nussbaum, Martha. (1990). *Love's knowledge: Essays on philosophy and literature*. New York: Oxford University Press.

Odent, Michel. (1981). The evolution of obstetrics at Pithiviers. *Birth and the Family Journal*, 1:8, 7–15.

O'Hara, Georgina. (1989). *The world of the baby. A celebration of infancy through the ages*. New York: Doubleday.

Olson, Carol. (1993). *The life of illness: One woman's journey*. New York: State University of New York Press.

Pagels, Elaine. (1989). *Adam, Eve, and the serpent*. New York: Vintage Books.

Parry, Alan, & Robert Doan. (1994). *Story re-visions: Narrative therapy in the postmodern world*. New York: The Guilford Press.

Paulette, Leslie. (1993). A choice for K'aila. *Humane Medicine*, 9:1, 13–17.

Peperzak, Adriaan. (1989). From intentionality to responsibility: On Levinas's philosophy of language. In Arleen B. Dallery & Charles E. Scott (Eds.), *The Question of the Other* (pp. 3–21). New York: State University of New York Press.

Piaget, Jean. (1952). *The origins of intelligence in children*. New York: International Press.

Piercy, Marge. (1991). *He, she and it*. New York: Alfred A. Knopf.

Polanyi, Michael. (1969). *Knowing and being*. Chicago: University of Chicago Press.

Portenier, Giselle. (Producer). (1994). Let her die. In J. Tufford (Producer), *Witness*. Toronto: Canadian Broadcasting Corporation.

Rabuzzi, Kathryn. (1988). *Motherself: A mythic analysis of motherhood*. Bloomington: Indiana University Press.

Rabuzzi, Kathryn. (1994). *Mother with child: Transformations through childbirth*. Bloomington: Indiana University Press.

Rapp, Rayna. (1984). XYLO: A true story. In R. Arditti, R. Duelli, & S. Minden (Eds.), *Test-tube Women* (pp. 313–328). Boston: Pandora Press.

Raymond, Janice G. (1990). Reproductive gifts and gift giving: The altruistic woman. *Hasting Center Report*, 20: 6, 7–11.

Reddy, Maureen T., Martha Roth, & Amy Sheldon. (Eds.). (1994). *Mothering journeys: Feminists write about mothering*. Minneapolis: Spinster Ink.

Resnick, Michael D., Robert W. Blum, Jane Bose, Martha Smith, & Roger Toogood. (1990). Characteristics of unmarried adolescent mothers: Determinants of childrearing versus adoption. *American Journal of Orthopsychiatry*, 60, 577–584.

Rich, Adrienne. (1976). *Of women born*. New York: Bantam Books.

Roberts, January, & Diane C. Robie. (1981). *Open adoption and open placement*. Brooklyn Park, Minn.: Adoption Press.

Rosenberg, Elinor B., & Thomas M. Horner. (1991). Birthparent romances and identity formation in adopted children. *American Journal of Orthopsychiatry*, 6:1, 70–77.

Ross, Jane. (1985). Musu's choice: An ethnography of perinatal care among the Kuranko of Sierra Leone. Unpublished doctoral dissertation. University of Cambridge, U.K.

Rothman, Barbara Katz. (1987). *Tentative pregnancy*. New York: Penguin.

Rothman, Barbara Katz. (1989). *Recreating motherhood: Ideology and technology in patriarchal society*. New York: W. W. Norton & Company.

Rothman, Barbara Katz. (1994). Beyond mothers and fathers: Ideology in a patriarchal society. In E. N. Glenn, G. Chang, & L. R. Forcey (Eds.), *Mothering. Ideology, experience, and agency* (pp. 139–157). London: Routledge.

Royal Commission on New Reproductive Technologies (Canada). (1991). *What we heard: Issues and questions raised during the public hearings*. Ottawa: The Commission.

Ruddick, Sara. (1983). Maternal thinking. In J. Trebilcot (Ed.), *Mothering: Essays in feminist theory* (pp. 211–230). Totowa, N.J.: Rowman & Allanhead.

Ruddick, Sara. (1989). *Maternal thinking: Toward a politics of peace*. Boston: Beacon Press.

Ryan, Kristapher. (1990). *From we to just me. A birth mother's journey: Decision-making, letting go, grieving, healing*. Winnipeg: Freedom to Be Me Seminars.

Sachdev, Paul. (1991). Achieving openness in adoption: Some critical issues in policy formulation. *American Journal of Orthopsychiatry, 61*, 241–249.

Sacks, Oliver. (1984). *A leg to stand on*. New York: Summit Books.

Sandelowski, Margarete. (1993). *With child in mind: Studies of the personal encounter with infertility*. Philadelphia: University of Pennsylvania Press.

Sandelowski, Margarete. (1994). We are the stories we tell: Narrative knowing in nursing practice: *Journal of Holistic Nursing, 12*:1, 23–33.

Sandelowski, Margarete, Betty G. Harris, & Diane Holditch-Davis. (1989). Mazing: Infertile couples and the quest for a child. *Image: Journal of Nursing Scholarship, 21*, 220–226.

Sandelowski, Margarete, Betty G. Harris, & Diane Holditch-Davis. (1993). "Somewhere out there." Parental claiming in the preadoption waiting period. *Journal of Contemporary Ethnography, 21*, 464–486.

Sarah, R. (1987). Power, certainty, and the fear of death. *Women & Health, 13*:1–2, 59–72.

Scarry, Elaine. (1985). *The body in pain: The making and unmaking of the world*. New York: Oxford University Press.

Scheper-Hughes, Nancy. (1992). *Death without weeping: The violence of everyday life in Brazil*. Berkeley: University of California Press.

Schluter, Andrea. (1994, May 6). It is a strange thing, the love of a mother. *Globe and Mail*, A20.

Schultz, Dawson, & Franco Carnevale. (1992). Engagement and suffering in responsible caregiving. Unpublished paper presented at the conference on The Empathetic Practitioner. Galveston, Texas. March.

Schweitzer, Ann. (1994). Exploring the narratives of relationship in intensive care nursing. Unpublished doctoral dissertation, University of Alberta.

Seiden, Anne. (1978). The sense of mastery in the childbirth experience. In M. Notman & C. Nadelson (Eds.). *The Woman Patient: Medical and Psychological Interfaces* (pp. 87–105). New York: Plenum Press.

Serey, A. M. (1992). The lived experience of being a teenage mother. Unpublished masters thesis: Florida Atlantic University.

Sherwin, Susan. (1992). *No longer patient: Feminist ethics & health care*. Philadelphia: Temple University Press.

Shuttle, Penelope, & Peter Redgrove. (1986). *The wise wound: Menstruation and everywoman*. London: HarperCollins Publishers.

Silko, Leslie Marmon. (1977). *Ceremony*. New York: Viking Press.

Simkin, Penny, Janet Whalley, & Ann Keppler. (1984). *Pregnancy, childbirth and the newborn: A complete guide for expectant parents*. Deephaven, Minn.: Meadowbrook.

Smith, David. (1984). The meaning of children in the lives of adults: A hermeneutic study. Unpublished doctoral dissertation. University of Alberta.

Smith, David. (1994). *Pedagon: Meditations on pedagogy and culture*. Bragg Creek, Alberta: Makyo Press.

SmithBattle, Lee. (1994). Beyond normalizing: The role of narrative in understanding teenage mothers' transition to mothering. In Patricia Benner (Ed.), *Interpretive phenomenology: Embodiment, caring and ethics in health and illness* (pp. 141–166). Thousand Oaks, Calif.: Sage Publications.

Sorel, Nancy. (1984). *Ever since Eve: Personal reflections on childbirth*. New York: Oxford University Press.

Sorosky, Arthur D., Annette Baran, & Reuben D. Pannor. (1978). *The adoption triangle: The effects of the sealed record on adoptees, birth parents, and adoptive parents*. Garden City, N.Y.: Anchor Press/Doubleday.

Spronk, Terri. (1992, September). Abandoning ownership: A philosophical approach to adoption. *Transition*, 6–7, 15.

Staples, David. (1995, September 22). Happiness is classified. *The Edmonton Journal*. A1.

Stolte, M. Mae. (1990). The nature and spirit of the birth archetype. Unpublished diploma thesis. C. G. Jung Institute, Zurich.

Swigart, Jane. (1991). *The myth of the bad mother: The emotional realities of mothering*. New York: Doubleday.

Tanner, Adrienne. (1993, August 20). Little David stays in B. C. *The Edmonton Journal*. A1.

Tennyson, Margaret S. (1988). Experiences of a woman who intended to relinquish her infant for adoption. *Maternal Child Nursing Journal*, 17:3, 139–152.

Tobey, Susan Bracaglia. (1991). *Art of motherhood*. New York: Abbeville Press, Inc.

Townsend, Rita, & Ann Perkins. (1992). *Bitter fruit: Women's experiences of unplanned pregnancy, abortion, and adoption*. Alameda, Calif.: Hunter House.

Triseliotis, John. (1973). *In search of origins: The experiences of adopted people*. London: Routledge & Kegan Paul.

van Manen, Max. (1990). *Researching lived experience: Human science for an action sensitive pedagogy*. London, Ontario: The Althouse Press.

Varela, Francisco, J., Evan Thompson, & Eleanor Rosch. (1991). *The embodied mind: Cognitive science and human experience*. Cambridge, Mass.: The MIT Press.

Victor, Lorraine, & Jane Persoon. (1994). Implementation of kangaroo care: A parent-health care team approach to practice change. *Critical Care Nursing Clinics of North America*, 6:4, 891–895.

Ward, Alison. (1993). Adoption, open. In B. K. Rothman (Ed.), *Encyclopedia of Childbearing: Critical Perspectives* (pp. 12–13). Phoenix, Ariz.: The Oryx Press.

Weizenbaum, J. (1976). *Computer power and human reason*. San Francisco: W. H. Freeman & Co.

Winkler, Robin, & Margaret van Keppel. (1984). *Relinquishing mothers in adoption: Their long-term adjustment*. Melbourne, Australia: Institute of Family Studies.

Woolf, Virginia. (1929). *A room of one's own*. New York: Fountain Press.

Young, Diony. (1987). Crisis in obstetrics: The management of labor. *International Journal of Childbirth Education*, 2:3, 13–15.

Young, Iris Marion. (1984). Pregnant embodiment: Subjectivity and alienation. *The Journal of Medicine and Philosophy*, 9:1, 45–60.

Index

About the Author

VANGIE BERGUM, Ph.D., is Professor in The Bioethics Centre and the Faculty of Nursing, University of Alberta. She is principal investigator of the Ethics of Nurturance Research Project which produced the video *and, they want a child* (University of Alberta, 1996). She is the author of numerous works, including *Woman to Mother: A Transformation* (Bergin & Garvey, 1989).

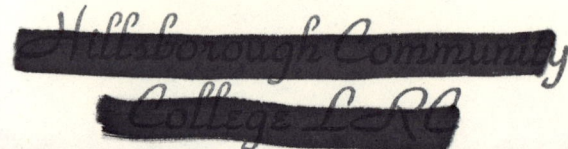